The Real You

ABOUT THE AUTHOR

After studying hypnotherapy, psychotherapy, coaching and a wide range of personal development techniques, Andrew Parr set up his own private practice to help people resolve personal, emotional and habitual problems. With nearly thirty years of experience, and having carried out over 17,000 one-to-one client consultations, he is one of the UK's most experienced hypnotherapists and personal-development coaches. He helps individuals and teams overcome limitations, and has his own practitioner academy based in East Sussex and online.

The Real You

How to Escape Your Limitations and Become the Person You Were Born to Be

ANDREW PARR

PENGUIN LIFE

AN IMPRINT OF

PENGUIN BOOKS

PENGUIN LIFE

UK | USA | Canada | Ireland | Australia
India | New Zealand | South Africa

Penguin Life is part of the Penguin Random House group of companies
whose addresses can be found at global.penguinrandomhouse.com.

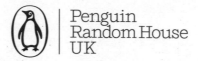

Penguin
Random House
UK

First published 2021
001

Copyright © Andrew Parr, 2021
Illustrations by Alice Parr, copyright © Andrew Parr, 2021

The moral right of the copyright holder has been asserted

Set in 12/14.75 pt Dante MT Std
Typeset by Jouve (UK), Milton Keynes
Printed and bound in Great Britain by Clays Ltd, Elcograf S.p.A.

The authorized representative in the EEA is Penguin Random House Ireland,
Morrison Chambers, 32 Nassau Street, Dublin D02 YH68

A CIP catalogue record for this book is available from the British Library

ISBN: 978–0–241–45353–7

www.greenpenguin.co.uk

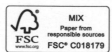

For my parents who gave their lives, to you, dear reader,
and to all the other everyday heroes

Contents

Contents

List of Exercises

Why Are You Here?

- Would you like to feel better about yourself, have greater self-confidence, increased self-worth and higher self-esteem, without becoming egotistical?
- Would you like to feel safer, more secure in the world, without having to overprotect yourself or shut yourself away?
- Would you like to feel stronger, more powerful, more in control of your life and the world around you, without needing to be overcontrolling of yourself or others?
- Would you like to feel that you have a unique place and purpose in this world, accepted and included, a sense of connection, without needing to change who you are?
- Would you like to experience more love and pleasure in your relationships without having to make sacrifices or experience loss in the process?
- Would you like to feel lighter and freer, more able to just be yourself?

If you can answer yes to any or all of these questions, this book is for you.

Dedicated to anyone who has ever struggled and to anyone who has ever dared to dream of something more, this book will give you an understanding of where your problems come from and why they may have been difficult to solve until now. Applied with honesty and persistance, my step-by-step set of exercises will help you make significant progress in improving conditions in each of the key areas of your life.

Caveat

This book is not intended to replace any kind of medical or therapeutic intervention. If you are suffering with a mental health condition or any form of Complex Post-Traumatic Stress Disorder (C-PTSD) you should seek the relevant professional help.

Introduction

It is 10.30 p.m. as I make my way on to the southbound platform of the Victoria Line at Oxford Circus underground station, London. There are only two other commuters on the platform, both male. Standing wide apart from each other, the first hasn't ventured much further than the passenger entrance and so is halfway along the platform. The other is way down near the opening of the tunnel where the trains emerge. I position myself midway between the two, as men do, half amused at myself for doing so.

As I hear a train approach, I glance left and see the lights coming down the tunnel and the man standing on the platform there. Just before the train emerges, I glance to my right to check the time, wondering if I will make the connection at Victoria.

An instant later I jolt back as an ear-splitting screech fills the tunnel. Covering my ears, I crouch back, sparks flying from the tracks as the speeding tube train attempts an emergency stop. When it finally comes to a standstill, only two-thirds out of the tunnel, there is an eery silence.

'Oh my God, did you see that, did you see that?' says the guy standing in the middle of the platform. 'He jumped, he jumped!'

I look left and, indeed, the man by the tunnel opening has disappeared, leaving just the two of us on the platform.

The train's doors remain locked, keeping the passengers inside, and for a minute or so there is further silence.

Eventually the platform staff arrive but, bizarrely, they completely ignore the other commuter and I, as if we are invisible. Nobody speaks to us, nobody asks us anything. We take a seat on the platform next to each other and watch in silence as the staff evacuate the train and guide the passengers out of the station. When the platform is finally clear, we are still sitting there, bemused by what has just happened. The two of us, a silent train, a few staff and a person – or body – somewhere on the track.

I exchange a few words with my fellow witness and then, realizing this route is now closed and the staff seem disinterested in our presence, I head out of the station and jump into a taxi to complete my connection at Victoria and make my way home.

What had caused him to jump? What was he running away from? What was he trying to do?

One of the most common reasons people commit suicide is an attempt to escape what they are feeling or experiencing and because they can see no positive viable future. Oddly, looking back now, at the time of this incident I completely understood how he may have been feeling. I say 'may' because it is actually impossible to know his motivations. But at this particular time in my life I was feeling stuck, trapped, even wanting the world to fall into chaos so I didn't have to face or deal with what I was going through. I'll share the details later but, not for the first time in my life, I understood why so many people want to bail out.

Each day feeling torn apart inside, I too wanted to escape. But not from life – I know the terrible damage that can leave behind for others and so have never seen that as an option. What I wanted to escape from was what I was feeling so that I could get on with life.

Many, many people reach that desperation point and of course there are occasions where a change of circumstances may be in order (we will cover that later), but this book is not about encouraging anyone to run away from anything. Ultimately, I don't believe we can – wherever we go we just take ourselves with us. It is especially not about encouraging anyone to run away from feelings and emotions because I do not believe we can do that either, though many people try.

This book is about escaping, resolving or overcoming our limitations – or perceived limitations – so that we can feel better now and move on in life. When we do that, new opportunities and new possibilities become available; things begin to change and we feel different. We make different choices, have different experiences, and tend to have, be and do more of what brings us greater satisfaction, pleasure, reward and happiness – and that is what I want you to experience more of by reading this book.

On the platform that evening, three strangers were drawn together; one ended his life, one I have no idea about, and the other – me – decided to put his life back together – again!

It wasn't easy and I did have to dig very, very deep at times, drawing upon resources that I hope my children never have to. But, having been to the metaphorical edge more than once over the years, I know that, however difficult it may seem, there is always a way back and it is always worth it.

The only character trait I believe I have that may have helped, and which I would encourage you to nurture in yourself, is that I am persistent.

Persistence has helped me with clients too. I didn't realize this until students repeatedly commented on it when watching me do live demos in front of the class at my Practitioner Academy. It seems that long after others would have given up or accepted at face value what was presented to them, I was still digging, encouraging the clients to probe deeper into the ideas causing a particular issue so that we could root them out at the cause. Deep and lasting change often requires patience and persistence, along with refusing to accept things at face value.

'Can you find this piece of Lego for me?' said my youngest son a few minutes ago as I was typing this. 'It's not there,' he said.

'What's it like?' I asked. He showed me the picture and I pretended to look as it was too small for me to see. 'It will be there somewhere, you will find a way. Look again in a different way,' I said, eager to return to my work. He huffed at me slightly and then found the missing piece a few moments later.

'You will find a way' is a phrase I have tried to drum into my children to help set them up for their own lives, probably because I have had to say it to myself more times than I care to mention. The same applies to you in whichever situation you currently find yourself. There is always a way.

The methods I am going to share with you are based upon my own experiences of working with many thousands of clients over the years, plus thousands of hours of teaching this to others and, of course, tackling my own foibles along the way.

After my life had somewhat fallen apart previously in my mid-twenties (which I will also expand on later), I one day found myself sitting on the floor of the run-down flat I was living in above a noisy and smelly kebab shop in North London. 'What am I going to do?' I asked, head in hands, to no one in particular. Which is when I heard a voice in my head say, 'Find out about hypnosis! Find out about hypnosis!'

So I did. Years before, I had seen a stage hypnotist on TV and also attended a live show at a college, but as I delved into the therapeutic side I became fascinated by the subject, the workings of the human mind and the potential for change. I studied hypnotherapy and psychotherapy, attended a variety of courses, read whatever books I could get my hands on (it was the Dark Ages then, no internet!) and eventually set up in private practice, aged just twenty-seven. People have often said to me how brave or courageous I was to do so at such a young age, but it wasn't that at all – it just never entered into my mind that I couldn't!

Hypnotherapy is pretty much divided into two main categories: clinical hypnosis and hypno-analysis. Clinical hypnosis tends to be very solution-focused, aimed at helping you bring about a solution by introducing a new idea into your mind via hypnotic suggestion, and there are many ways of applying that; in contrast, hypno-analysis (sometimes called analytical hypnosis) aims to resolve the underlying causes. In fact, the whole world of therapy is often divided and subdivided in this way, and factions can become quite religious about the pros and cons of each, largely, I believe, owing to whichever branch they were introduced to when they began to study. I was lucky enough to have been introduced to both solution-focused and analytical approaches, so have always been able to see the benefits of each, and switch between them where appropriate, as well as drawing in elements from a whole range of other specializations.

However, I have never really liked being called a therapist, hypnotherapist, coach or anything like that – actually, I have never liked labels, full stop. I have always enjoyed solving problems and puzzles and this is how I would like to encourage you to consider any situation in life you are seeking to change or transform, right now: as a puzzle to solve.

Whatever you are going through or whichever limitations you would like to be free of, please be assured there is always a way – we just need to figure out which piece of the puzzle is creating the problem for you and put your mind to work at that level.

I have often looked at people who have beaten the odds, overcome difficulties or achieved success in an endeavour and said to myself, 'Well, if they can do it, so can I.' Flipping that around now, the same is true for you: if I can do it – and still am – you can too. You just need to be persistent in the right way – and to not be afraid of facing up to a few things.

Anyone can do that, right? Because if you can, everything else takes care of itself.

Although I will often refer to hypnosis throughout this book, this is not a book about hypnotherapy. It is about helping you to transform your life, and there are many tools I have used to assist people with that. But it is important to remember that it is not so much the achievement of goals or overcoming our struggles in itself that brings us the satisfaction we are looking for. It is the *personal growth and transformation* we go through in making the attempt that really matters. It is not even the old 'journey versus the destination' idea, but more about the person we *become* on that journey. That is the real prize here, that is the gem.

The goal itself will eventually lose its shine or novelty; the person we have to become to get there can endure.

When I was seventeen I attended a lecture by entrepreneur and philanthropist John James, who was a benefactor to the school I attended in Bristol (thanks to a fee-assistance programme as it would otherwise have been beyond my parents' means). I usually dozed through such lectures but this one in particular made a deep and lasting impression. 'My goal in life has always been to be healthy, wealthy and wise – in that order,' said James in a very humble and unassuming manner.

It was the 'in that order' that got my attention. 'Health is a priority,' he explained, 'as without health, everything else takes on less meaning,' or words to that effect. Wealth would enable him to enjoy life and do good in the world, he went on, and he would rather be wealthy and stupid than wise but poor, which made me smile! Wisdom would be a nice bonus, but if not, he would at least have been healthy and enjoyed his life, while being able to help others in the process. To me it seemed a worthy goal or ideal and, for whatever reason, those words and James's voice have stayed with me my whole life, quietly reassuring me when I felt a little lost or unsure of myself, inspiring me when I needed a kick from behind.

If you are reading this book you *will* have a goal, right now, whether you realize it or not. Your goal will most likely be to transform how you are thinking, feeling or behaving in some area of life in order to achieve a certain outcome that means something to you.

You will have an issue – what I call a 'surface-level symptom' – that you want to change, ease or remove and replace with something that makes you feel better. You will want to stop thinking, feeling, doing or experiencing one thing and start thinking, feeling, doing or experiencing something else.

The pain or discomfort of the surface-level symptom will be the motivator for you to take action; the *person you become* on the journey to resolving that surface-level symptom is what will actually set you free and make you happier.

What most people do not yet fully realize is the extent to which we are each battling against ourselves, and only by addressing both our conscious and subconscious thoughts, feelings and emotions around a particular issue can we truly get from where we are to where we want to be – *and stay there*. Any attempt at change without addressing these and any emotive forces behind them will otherwise always be temporary or leave us with the feeling of trying to run up a down escalator. Having tried this late one night on one of the longest escalators in the London Underground, I can assure you it is very tiring. We get so far on willpower and enthusiasm alone, but after a while we find ourselves running merely to stand still. Eventually we tire and end up back at the bottom where we started, with the top looking a long way up. Feeling disheartened or jaded by the experience, we may then be tempted to put off further attempts for some time.

Sound familiar?

With that in mind, this book is *not* about having more willpower and determination to keep running up that down escalator until we make it to the top (though willpower and determination are very important when used in the right way). This book is more about what makes it a down escalator in the first place and what we can do to ease and reverse this effect so that it becomes one which can then carry us in the direction we wish to travel more easily.

For example, when jet skier Paul Hewitt came to see me, he told me he was having trouble performing a certain trick he wanted to incorporate into the routine he was developing for an upcoming competition. The trick involved taking his 800cc jet ski through a very tight 180-degree turn, which gave him the momentum he needed to submerge the jet ski vertically, nose pointing upward. As the jet ski sank down, he wanted to leap from the sitting position so that his hands went on to the nose, while his feet jumped on to the handles so that his foot could operate the throttle. Then, with the jet ski reaching its lowest point underwater and his foot holding the throttle on full power as long as possible, Paul wanted to 'monkey jump' on to the nose so that as the jet ski picked up speed and fired out of the water like a rocket, it did so with Paul on the nose in a handstand position!

'I keep holding back at the crucial moment,' he told me, and I looked at him incredulously, wondering how sane this very likeable, mild-mannered man was.

However, when we delved into it, identifying the precise fear going through his mind at the crucial moment, we uncovered a pattern of holding himself back that had played itself out through many areas of his life.

As we resolved that fear, Paul found a new level of confidence: not only did he pull off the trick beautifully, right in front of the judges, but his performance enabled him to win the British Freestyle Jet Ski Championship title outright that weekend, with a final round still to go. The release of the fear rippled out into other areas of life as well, allowing him to move on in so many different ways, and he now helps others do the same.

We may not all want to do handstands on jet skis, but the daily thoughts, feelings and emotions we experience, and the personal, emotional and habitual problems that arise from these when they trigger stress and anxiety, will cause us to have issues that hold us back. Some will be obvious; some will be much more subtle. And often the attempt to alleviate these issues will cause further issues, as we will discover.

Some people just live with this and accept it as the way they are and the way life is. Others seek help from a professional therapist – and I use that term to cover the many forms of talky and non-talky therapies available. Others, still, turn to the plethora of self-help books on offer.

Therapy can be extremely beneficial and transformative for many people, but for others it can take a very long time to make little, if any, real progress, especially where the deeper, more ingrained issues are concerned. Many clients coming to me from long-term therapy have told me they have an excellent understanding of their issue, but they still have the issue!

Self-help books can be incredibly informative, inspiring and trans-formative, and have no doubt saved countless lives and helped countless more. But at times they can also be oversimplistic or make personal development sound too easy.

Let's face it, self-help is often difficult; therapy is often difficult. It doesn't need to be, but it often is. There is a solution, however, which we will discuss later in the book.

Most people seeking my help over the years have asked me to give them something – more confidence, more calmness, more control, more willpower, more inner strength, more determination – to stop thinking, feeling or behaving the way they have been and start thinking, feeling and behaving in a different way. But I have found that the most effective way to really help someone long-term is to first take something away – it may be a false idea, an invisible belief, a self-imposed limitation – and then allow it to be replaced by something more positive. This book, therefore, is about taking you on a journey to the core of your perceived fears and limitations, facing any raw emotions that are lurking there and coming back renewed, refreshed and, most importantly, released.

Every time I do this, or help to do this, with a client I see the person grow and become something more. More themselves. More authentic. More real. More free.

For the main part, then, I have actually spent most of my time helping people undo what has happened to them or, more accurately, undo the limiting ideas and beliefs they have collected through what has happened to them, which later manifest as blocks, challenges or dysfunctional attitudes and behaviours.

In a way, we can say that each of us has been hypnotized by life. Using the clichéd view of hypnosis, life has introduced ideas into our minds that we now accept as truth and act on accordingly, sometimes consciously, sometimes subconsciously, which can bring about both positive and negative changes in our behaviour and hence in our life. Each time we have accepted an idea as 'truth' without necessarily challenging it or testing it, we can say that life has programmed us using a process of nat-ural hypnosis.

When we use this phenomenon for our benefit, it adds to our life. When we use it against ourselves, problems occur. Very often, without realizing, while we are consciously desiring of one thing, we are unconsciously focusing on something else. This was the case in our jet ski example earlier, with Paul wanting to complete a trick but an old idea holding him back, until we were able to resolve it.

It is the conflict between the two that causes the problem – and that conflict will be largely owing to invisible or unchallenged ideas within us. But using naturally occurring states of mind we can tap into the realm where the conflicting ideas are operating and begin to make deeper and more lasting changes at the causative level.

On a training course recently I invited Olympic kayak bronze medalist Ian Wynne to demonstrate a new technology ProCVT, developed by ProBiometrics, which uses extremely accurate measurements of changes in heart rate to determine vagal tone. He explained that our hearts' natural tempo is around 110 beats per minute but the vagus nerve puts a brake on the heart to slow it down to what we measure as the usual, everyday restful rate.

However, in times of stress or danger or when we need extra energy, the vagus nerve releases the brake. The heart almost instantly returns to its higher rate, which is much more effective and efficient than ramping up gradually.

In a similar way, I have always seen it as my job to *dehypnotize* people, to release their brakes. I am a dehypnotizer who helps people release their psychological, emotional and physiological brakes, often by helping them access emotionally charged memories or ideas that have been causing the false beliefs deep within them.

Having observed this occur in my clients thousands of times over the years, however, I have also grown to realize something else: on our journey through life, underneath the layers of doubt and limitation we tend to pick up, is what I have come to call the 'Real You' waiting to shine through. This Real You actually has good self-worth, feels safe and secure in the world, is in control of their life, feels accepted and has the ability to form loving relationships.

It has also slowly dawned on me over the years that every attempt to alleviate a surface-level symptom is actually an attempt to take us one step closer to becoming more of our real selves – or allowing more of that part of our identity to come to the surface. And every time we allow ourselves to operate from the perspective of our real self, life feels good or gets better in some way. And, conversely, when we don't it feels bad or gets worse.

But . . . I need to make it clear it isn't just about *getting rid* of all the 'bad stuff'; I have also observed through my clients and myself that the 'bad stuff' matters, is valid, and actually adds to our life. It gives us something that we wouldn't have had without it. Although it may seem like a limitation or painful experience while going through it, in the overcoming of it we have the opportunity to grow and become something more.

If there was an equation it would be:

Real You + Overcoming Limitations = Something More

That 'something more' is what I call 'The Person You Were Born to Be'!

The Person You Were Born to Be is a more evolved version of what you would otherwise have been had you not encountered those difficulties and limitations in life in order to grow and *become* that person.

So if there are any areas where you currently feel stuck, are struggling or unable to make significant progress right now, please do not despair. Each of these is offering an opportunity for growth in a very practical, life-transforming way that extends far beyond the surface-level symptoms that drove you to seek help in the first place.

I am not saying it is easy and I am not saying that you can do it all on your own. Having spent nearly thirty years hypnotically exploring the workings of the human mind, this book is a summary of what I have learned so far about helping people; about what you can do yourself and what you may need some help with, and why, though not necessarily from a paid professional. This book is actually, therefore, more of a bridge between self-help and therapy, a gap that has been in need of filling for a long time.

One of the challenges of writing this book, however, was how to translate the deeply moving and transformational experience of an intimate one-to-one session – taking the client on a journey deep within themselves, peeling away layers of fear and limitation, then bringing them back renewed and refreshed, with a new perspective on themselves and life – into a set of self-help exercises. If at times the exercises seem complex, therefore, it is only because we as humans tend to make things so, and the exercises are designed to peel away that complexity. Underneath it all, the answer is always very, very simple.

I know you have been through difficulties that have created limitations in your life; I know there is a Real You within, waiting to be released. If I can help you identify any self-imposed limitations you have been carrying within you – both known and unknown – and make progress at overcoming them, then I believe you can and will become even more of the Person You Were Born to Be and experience greatly improved conditions in your life, with greater levels of reward, happiness and personal satisfaction.

Although trained in hypnotherapy and psychotherapy, I have also dipped into the worlds of coaching, counselling, NLP, personal development and most areas of teaching where there is a possibility of helping someone change. As a result, I have developed my own system – the E.S.C.A.P.E. Method – that will help to dehypnotize you from what no longer serves you and instead allow a more evolved version of the Real You to shine through.

If you feel that now is the time for you to evolve to the next level of your being, then let's begin. As I always teach my students, though, 'First seek to understand, then seek to resolve,' otherwise how do we know we are trying to resolve the right thing? So let's start by taking a closer look at that.

PART ONE

Why We Have Problems and What They Really Are

Models of the Mind

Before we can even begin to think about resolving problems or understand what I mean by dehypnotizing, we need to understand how life hypnotizes us in the first place and how that creates problems, repeating cycles, generally making life difficult at times. Only then can we truly bring about a lasting solution. Only then can we not only solve problems and break repeating patterns and cycles, but also evolve in some way.

There are two main Models of the Mind I use when explaining this. I initially came across a basic version of the first one, which I refer to as the Pyramid Model, when attending a course on stress management many years ago, though I have adapted it and renamed it since. The second, which I refer to as the Library Model, is one I created for the first-ever training course I ran, and I developed the diagram as students asked questions, based on my observations of working with clients.

The Pyramid Model

Most of us are familiar with the terms 'conscious' and 'subconscious' (or 'unconscious') mind, but I am going to explain these in a slightly different way that you may not yet be familiar with, as it can sometimes feel as if these are two different entities or personalities, battling away within us.

The conscious part of our mind represents anything that we are consciously aware of in any particular moment. As you are reading this you may be aware of the book or device you are reading from or indeed listening to. You may also be aware of what is happening in your immediate surroundings, such as the air temperature if it is meaningful to you (it is a little chilly where I am right now and part of my thoughts are thinking about switching on the heating). You may also be aware of the chair/sofa/bed/beach/train/bath/grass or whatever is supporting your body at this moment, as well as any sounds you can hear and possibly even a vague thought about something you may need to be doing later on.

Although you know your name, where you live and other such information, these are probably not in your conscious awareness until I mention them. But now that I have, they probably are, and as a result some of the other thoughts such as what you are doing later may have had to give way to make space. But now I have mentioned them again they will be back once more and your name will have slipped away. Wait, it's back!

This short-term processing of information is often referred to as our 'working memory' and we generally say that the conscious mind can handle around four or five pieces of information at any one time, though this can be more for some people, less for others. Without wishing to create gender stereotypes, studies have shown that women, it seems, can do slightly better than men when it comes to multi-processing verbal information.

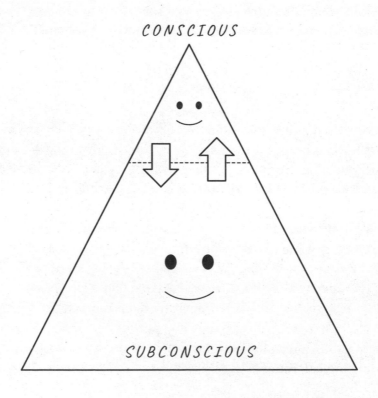

Talk to me while I am watching a movie and I will look at you with irritation. I can talk to you – or I can watch a movie – but please don't ask me to do both, that would be crazy.

However, when we talk about the spatial awareness processing aspect of working memory, which includes visualization and navigation, some studies suggest that males tend to find this easier than females. Overall performance, though, seems to balance out, so best not get too hung up on this in case we try to live up to stereotypes!

The main point I wish to get across is that the conscious part of our mind is designed to carry only a limited quantity of information at any one time that we can focus on and apply logic to and we are constantly moving information into and out of our conscious awareness, depending on *what we deem is important and worthy of our attention.* (Pay attention to that last part of the sentence.)

In the working memory model, the decision about what is important for the conscious mind to focus on is handled by the area known as the 'central executive'. 'Should I continue talking to my friend or should I pause for a moment and divert resources to assess how safe it is to cross the road?' is a typical decision the central executive will make.

What happens to detail like our name and address when we are not consciously needing it? It is of course stored somewhere below our everyday awareness but still accessible and we usually call this the sub-conscious or unconscious. 'Sub' means under or beneath, whereas 'un' means not, and although I tend to use the two interchangeably, for the purposes of this book I will use subconscious, meaning under or beneath our full conscious awareness. With this in mind, the first main point I want you to be aware of here is that information can flow back and forth between our conscious and subconscious awareness, depending upon what we deem is important to focus on at any one time. Let's now take a quick look at some of the functions of each in practice.

Functions

The conscious part of our mind is designed for focused attention, including logical, rational decision-making and very deliberate, aware, strategic-thinking processes. The subconscious takes care of pretty much everything else.

The conscious mind will help us look at a bus timetable and calculate what time we need to get somewhere and which bus to catch and what time we have to leave in order to do so. The subconscious mind will help us remember what a bus is, what we can expect to happen, what it feels like to be on it, plus keep our body alive, breathing and functioning while we do.

The subconscious mind has many functions, but for the purposes of this chapter I would like to draw your attention to its ability to store and retrieve information, and the impact that has on each of us.

Consider what happens as we go through life. Let's say there is an event – something happens. We sit on a chair for the first time; we hold a pen; we lean on a table; we drink from a cup. Each of these events makes an impression which we store as a memory that is then available for recall later on when we need it, usually in response to some kind of trigger.

This is great because it means that we do not have to learn everything new each time we encounter it. It means that we can walk into a room we have never been into before and see objects we have never seen before, yet know what they are.

Our mind receives incoming information via our senses, checks around inside for what we know about that information and then sends a message up to our conscious awareness so that we know what we are dealing with and have an idea of what to do.

It's a pen, I can write with it.

It's a table, I can place things on it.

It's a cup, I can drink from it.

I have never seen that exact pen/table/cup before but it fits the general look and feel of what I know about things that look like that so I am assuming that's what it is.

We take it for granted, but this process is occurring every moment that we are awake – a constant receiving of input, referencing inside for what we know, followed by a response as to how we should proceed. Various studies have estimated that we have around 60,000 or more thoughts each day.

Can you imagine how complicated life would be if every day we had to discover what everything was, as if encountering it for the very first time? Thank goodness we have this learning system to make it easier.

However . . . let's add an extra dimension to make this a little more interesting. Pens, tables and cups are very useful but are unlikely to make deep and lasting impressions unless out of the ordinary. So let's bring in some feelings and emotions.

When I was eleven years old I used to take a fifty-minute bus ride to and from school and it was nearly always the same: same time, same bus, same route each day. One day, there were problems on my usual return route so I took a different bus which dropped me about a mile from home and I planned to walk the rest of the way through the park. As I stepped into the park, however, I saw an unaccompanied dog ahead of me, blocking the path. At this time in my life, I had never really encountered dogs close up, save for a few visits to distant family members with dogs, but dogs were always scary for me. Unpredictable beasts with lots of teeth, scratchy claws and panty breath; all in all, potentially dangerous and unpleasant creatures, best to be avoided.

The fear and panic I felt were almost as if it were a lion stood there. I tried to tell myself it was OK, but fear got the better of me and I ended up backing out of the park and taking the most ridiculous detour home, arriving an hour or so later than expected, doing my best to hold back tears following the close encounter with death I had narrowly escaped. Or so I felt.

The memory of this experience stayed with me for years and the feeling 'dogs are dangerous, might chase me and bite me' triggered mistrust and anxiety whenever I was close to one. Any time I saw a roaming dog, somewhere in my mind I was transported back to that moment in the park, and this continued almost up until the day I got my own dogs (two Tibetan terriers, which are the closest thing I know to living teddy bears). And all the poor dog back then had done was stand there and look at me!

If we experience something that creates a strong feeling or emotion, we not only create a memory of that, we also, in a way, wrap that memory in the associated feeling or emotion.

Then, when something comes along that triggers that memory, we are quite likely to experience the same feeling or emotion as well. A photograph that brings back fond memories of a holiday; a familiar smell that

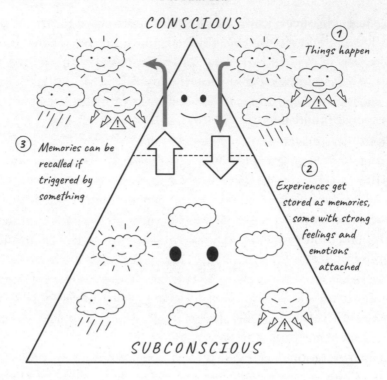

CONSCIOUS

① Things happen

③ Memories can be recalled if triggered by something

② Experiences get stored as memories, some with strong feelings and emotions attached

SUBCONSCIOUS

transports us back to a pleasant scene; or a dog that reminds us of being scared in the park.

Something happens, it triggers something inside, and we have an experience.

Now, in very, very simple terms, this is what is happening with any of us who have a specific issue caused by a specific past experience or set of experiences. Something happens whereby our senses receive incoming information, and this creates an emotional response.

Think of something unpleasant that has happened in your life. How quickly are you able to bring it to mind, or even begin to feel a little (or a lot) of what you were feeling back then? Sometimes very easily, sometimes not so, but the same process is occurring: if something comes along that triggers a memory with an unpleasant or uncomfortable feeling wrapped around it, we will most likely experience some or all of that emotion in that moment of remembering as well.

But that is not all. The emotional response then makes us want to either do or not do something; if we have a fear, such as dogs, injections, people or public speaking, for example, if we cannot challenge it then we typically want to run, hide, escape or avoid it.

Now, it is important to realize that we do not consciously choose or decide to have whichever feeling is triggered – it often seems to 'just happen'. Feeling anxious, tense or scared may appear out of our control as if the response is *automatic*. But it only seems to be automatic because we are not fully conscious of the whole process. The subconscious part is hidden or tucked away – under or out of our awareness. It doesn't mean it is not happening, it just means we are not consciously aware of it happening, usually because it is so fast. While it takes up to 500ms (half a second) for our conscious mind to make sense of a situation, our subconscious can respond in just 12ms, or in the case of a loud noise, just 5ms – that's one hundred times faster than we can consciously think, which could save our lives in a potentially threatening situation, such as helping us to jump back at a startling sound.

The result is that information comes in and our subconscious processes work beautifully, delivering a near-instantaneous response based on its interpretation of the information.

What's interesting is the subsequent effect on us. Our natural inclination in the future is, of course, to try to avoid the source of the fear or unpleasant feeling, whatever it may be. So, using our examples from above, we may try to avoid dogs, injections, people or speaking in public. Which makes sense, right?

Except, unfortunately, it doesn't work like that. The strange thing is, it seems that ultimately we cannot avoid these things. We cannot simply avoid the source of our fears or limitations or whatever issues we may be going through because something within us seems to seek them out – or attract them – or both. We seem to draw towards us – or draw ourselves towards – the very things we want to avoid. Whatever we fear or dread will pop up, again and again. We seem to be drawn to it like a magnet.

The person with a fear of dogs will encounter dogs everywhere; the person with a fear of injections will need blood tests or travel inoculations; the person with a fear of speaking in public will find themselves in a role that demands speaking in front of a group from time to time.

How this happens, we'll discuss later, but for now I want you to be aware that *whatever we carry within us, and give enough energy, emotion or focus to, finds a way to express itself.* And the more we try to resist this, the more it seems to persist!

When these persist over a period of time, repeating patterns develop. Patterns of thoughts, feelings and behaviours. The external characters and situations in our life may change, but the thoughts, feelings and behaviours they create will be unnervingly familiar.

And here's the sting. As we experience old feelings in new situations, these new situations get added to our existing store of information of how we think life is and thereby reinforce the old feelings and emotions. This then adds even more significance, meaning and emotional momentum to the process, causing us to further repeat this scenario, often throughout our lives, unless we find a way to end the cycle.

It is not just obvious fears that create this repeating cycle, but all feelings and emotions. For instance, someone with an abusive parent will often find themselves with abusive partners; someone bullied at school will find themselves bullied at work; someone made to feel guilt and shame when younger will find themselves doing things that lead to feelings of guilt and shame as an adult.

It can flip the other way as well. The young person who was made to feel weak and insignificant becomes overdominant and aggressive; a child who was shamed and put down becomes the shamer and criticizer of others; a young life filled with fear and violence may seek out the same when older, inflicting fear and violence on others.

I am giving you a simplified explanation here but I hope you get the idea.

The net result is that we form a loop, whereby whatever we hold inside seeks expression and brings more of the same back to us, creating experiences that push the same feelings and emotions to the surface, reinforcing the ideas that created them in the first place, which then create more.

These loops can be very difficult to break using conventional methods – especially if we are not even aware they are happening and just think, 'Oh no! Why me? Not again!' But these loops are what we must dissolve if we are to be free of our limitations and able to fully move on. These loops will be driven by emotionally charged ideas, both known and unknown, visible and invisible. When we can identify all the ideas at play concerning a particular issue and, most importantly, dissolve any emotional investment we have in them, the loops weaken and the repeating cycles reduce or cease entirely, as do the surface-level symptoms that were created by them.

Now, I am not saying that every event we experience that contains a negative feeling or emotion creates an issue and I am not saying that every issue we have comes about in this way. But if we have some kind of experience that creates a strong emotive response, often early in our lives, and that emotive response is not dealt with properly at the time and instead penetrates the subconscious mind, then *our subconscious mind will seek opportunities to keep us feeling the same way.* Not all the time, not every moment . . . but it will seek opportunities to do so until the issue is dealt with.

In this way, life hypnotizes us to think, feel or behave in certain ways at certain times, in exactly the same way that a stage hypnotist gets his or her subjects to respond to certain cues. We think we are going about our day running our own lives but, actually, most of us have been hypnotized by life so that at times we are merely responding to subconscious triggers and recreating patterns, the outcome of which we then have to do our best to try to deal with consciously.

The dichotomy, it seems then, is this: we simultaneously have both free will and yet are at the mercy of our subconscious programming from life. We are constantly moving into and out of different states of mind – sometimes exercising free will, sometimes merely responding to our programming.

When our conscious free will and our subconscious programming are aligned, things tend to go well and we feel good. But when our conscious free will and subconscious programming – from the ideas we carry inside – are in conflict, that is when we find ourselves struggling and trying to run up the down escalator.

And on top of that, it is as if there is some kind of inescapable process at work that is designed to bring us into close contact with *more and more* of these triggers, so that we each have our very own personal version of the world that knows exactly how to push the button on our individual fears and sensitivities. No wonder it feels difficult sometimes!

Beliefs Are Opinions, Not Fact

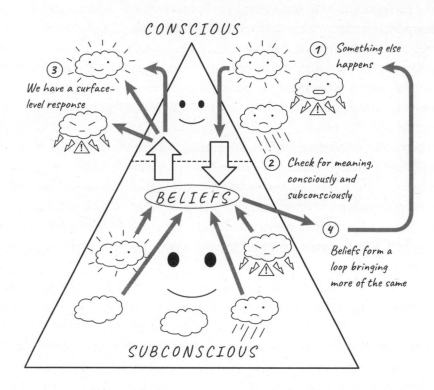

CONSCIOUS

① Something else happens

③ We have a surface-level response

② Check for meaning, consciously and subconsciously

BELIEFS

④ Beliefs form a loop bringing more of the same

SUBCONSCIOUS

As you can imagine, as we go through life we take in a lot of information and store it for future reference, so after a while our memory and information storage systems get pretty busy. It would be extremely inefficient if our mind had to go through every single memory of every single experience every single time we encountered something, simply to identify what it is and what we are supposed to do, so to speed up the process we have an easy referencing system, which we call our 'beliefs'.

We can say that our beliefs are a summary of everything we have learned about a certain subject or topic until this moment, so that when 'something happens', and our mind says, 'What do I know about this, and how should I respond?', we have some kind of reference and can react or respond accordingly, which may be especially important for our survival if facing a threat or danger.

Our beliefs may not necessarily be true or accurate! But they are what we *believe* to be true, based on our interpretation of our life experiences so far. We could say that beliefs are really just opinions, formed from our interpretation of the information available to us at a certain time; nevertheless, they cause us to seek out experiences and encounters that reinforce them, making them seem even more 'true'.

In our Mind Model, we can say that many of these beliefs sit just under our awareness, ready to be accessed when required, and they cover every area of our lives, including health, relationships, career and more. In fact, in any area where we have thoughts, feelings and emotions that lead to behaviours, our beliefs will be at play.

We have personal beliefs, family beliefs, cultural beliefs, spiritual and religious beliefs, organizational beliefs and societal beliefs, to name a few. And we have beliefs that cause our issues. Indeed, we can say that:

Our issues run as deep as our beliefs. No more. No less.

Yet I want to get away from the idea of them being buried deep and hard to access. From my experience, many of the ideas that cause us problems are actually very conscious and available for scrutiny, but we accept them so readily as 'the way things are', they seem invisible, making them difficult to spot – at first.

It is also important to realize that these beliefs cannot exist without a reason, and at some level of our mind we will have supporting evidence that makes them valid – usually emotive memories or experiences.

- 'I got stung by a bee when I was young so I now believe bees will hurt me.'
- 'I was told by a teacher I respected that I was useless at learning and so I now believe I am useless at learning.'
- 'I felt less important than my sibling, so I now believe I am less worthy of love and attention.'

But take a look at the end of each of those statements above and think about what the effect of each might be. If those thoughts are allowed to play out subconsciously next time we encounter the situations they would be saying . . .

- 'Bees will hurt me.'
- 'I am useless at learning.'
- 'I am less worthy of love and attention.'

Can you imagine how we would behave in certain circumstances if life had hypnotized us to believe these to be true? We would go into situations with these preconceived ideas and react accordingly if anything seemed to trigger them. We would quite possibly be on the alert and actively looking out for them, and on top of that, our mind would also somehow keep putting us in situations where we encountered them.

The net result is that we have a system whereby we store information, including feelings and emotions, that we can consciously and subconsciously reference at a later date if need be, via our beliefs, so that we know what to do or how to be. But that system also seems to want to repeat itself or keep us trapped in cycles, bringing more of the same issues into our lives that keep us feeling the same way!

Or does it?

You see, so far we have put the emphasis on what we usually describe as negative beliefs and experiences – things that make us feel bad, scared, stuck, lost, down, hurt and so on. But exactly the same principle applies for all the good stuff in our life as well.

Positive experiences can cause positive beliefs which help draw towards us – or draw us towards – experiences of what we perceive to be a positive nature: happy, safe, loved, fun, strong, successful and so on.

And what I have noticed over the years of helping people, as well as myself, is that every time we resolve or dissolve an old limiting belief, not only do the symptoms and repeating patterns which were coming from that begin to reduce, fade or disappear, but they are replaced by new, more positive versions – which then go on to create new 'symptoms' and repeating patterns, only this time of a more positive nature, loops we are usually quite happy to remain stuck in!

When an old tree topples, a new
sapling takes its place.

So instead of a system in which we are trapped by our limiting beliefs and experiences, it seems we actually have a system whereby we will repeat those same patterns of thoughts, feelings and behaviours, along with the outcomes they create, until such time as we choose to deal with the causes. At which time we evolve to a new level of experience – usually one that brings a greater sense of reward, freedom and happiness. And this system seems to *want* us to heal or evolve because it keeps providing the means and opportunity to do so!

Symptoms and Problems – Or Opportunities in Disguise?

If our mind – or life – seems to keep bringing things back to us, or putting us in situations where we feel the same way, there must be a reason. When studying nature and evolution, the little quirks and features the plants and creatures of this planet possess each serve a purpose in some way. They – we – have evolved over millions of years and nature tends to enhance the useful and do away with the not so useful.

So this human feature of repeating cycles of emotions and experiences, driven by our beliefs, must serve a purpose. Could it be, then, that this phenomenon of repeating cycles and patterns, or encountering 'negative' experiences driven by our beliefs, is actually part of an evolutionary process? It would certainly help us increase our chances of surviving danger by recognizing the signs early on so we can take action; but could it also be that the issues we perceive as symptoms and problems are actually *personal* evolutionary opportunities in disguise?

When I injured my back a while ago, I could barely move for nearly ten days. Going to the bathroom involved a half-hour shuffle with a walking stick, sometimes having to pause on the way if I moved too quickly, triggering spasms that made me tremble with the pain. I remember almost breaking down in tears of frustration one day at my helplessness as I couldn't figure out how to get my hand from the door handle that was supporting me to my daughter's shoulder, who was there to help me round a corner where there was nothing else to hold on to; I remember looking at a kettle, wondering how I would ever be able to make tea again because lifting such a heavy object seemed an insurmountable task. I remember the loss of dignity I felt at being wheeled around an airport in a wheelchair, suddenly gaining insight and empathy with those in a similar condition. 'Not so invincible and fiercely independent now, are you?' I remember thinking to myself, catching my reflection in a window, pride slipping away.

The message was very, very clear: instead of running around pushing myself to the limits, taking care of everybody else, I needed to slow down, learn to accept more help and take greater care of myself. As I recovered this time – because I had been through this before – something within me finally realized it was time to change or evolve. Using the methods described in this book as I faced up to the insecurities that had been driving me so hard in the first place, my needs and wants changed and evolved, and greater levels of happiness and satisfaction have followed.

The same can be true for any of our life situations. The breakdown of a relationship may cause us to face up to our inner issues that led to it, thereby paving the way for a more loving and satisfying experience next time. A repeated injury on the sports field may lead us to examine the drivers that created it, encouraging us to approach training and fitness in a more productive way, enabling consistently higher levels of performance when we return. 'Failure' in any area of life can make us question previously unexamined beliefs and values, so that we can finally achieve greater success.

This idea is not new – we have been reading it in novels and watching it in movies all of our lives, and the plot line is always the same. We begin by learning about the main character or characters, who are busy going about their lives. Then something happens that causes them to go on some kind of quest or journey. It usually starts off well at first and things seem to fall into place – something we may experience as 'beginner's luck'. But then something else happens. In a superhero movie, the supervillain appears. In our own more down-to-earth version, everything goes wrong, we experience failure, loss and helplessness, and, like our superhero, seem stripped of our power or ability to find a way forward. All hope is lost and we feel desperate.

But then something else happens. A way opens up. A new possibility arises often from the least expected source. But there is risk involved. We cannot remain as we were and survive. We have to change or evolve if we are to succeed and there is usually some sort of existential shift, leading to a 'do or die' moment when we have to fully commit. In a novel or a movie, that is the part where we buy into the character's dilemma and are with them as they face the ultimate challenge. There may be losses on the way – and what seem like sacrifices – but when the story is over and the battle is won, we are left changed by it. We are older, wiser, more evolved, and we then establish a new normal.

Recognize the story?

At first this can make the idea of change seem quite daunting – isn't it just easier and safer to stay as we are?

Perhaps . . . But, as we have mentioned, life also seems to have a habit of wanting us to evolve in some way – and however much we try to maintain our status quo, that 'something' happens . . . and we are forced on to the quest.

There is one thing that is very important for us to realize, however. The quest itself is not the problem – it is our *resistance* to it that causes the difficulties.

As we make our way through this book, I want you to understand that all of this is actually very, very simple, and that you already have everything you need to be able to make whatever changes you wish in life. A little self-examination and a dose of persistence will go a long way towards easing or transforming the unpleasant symptoms and conditions of our lives, and we'll be going through exercises to help with that later on.

Simple doesn't mean easy, however, and there will be some challenges we need to face. But if, from now on, we can begin to see these problems or challenges as opportunities in disguise, each carrying a hidden jewel presenting possibilities of personal transformation, then the challenges can become more palatable to deal with, as long as we know they are serving a purpose and there is something better waiting on the other side. And from personal experience, I would say that the sooner we start, the better, because otherwise our minds will have to go to greater and greater lengths to get our attention.

Each time we ease or resolve something in ourselves, it also has an impact on those around us. For example, as we finally feel greater self-worth, love and acceptance, it becomes easier to create or inspire that in others, which naturally makes our corner of the world a nicer place to be for us and those around us. Could it be that these so-called issues, symptoms and problems we face are not only creating opportunities in disguise at the individual level, but also thereby encouraging a form of emotional evolution for the species as a whole?

I'll leave you to ponder that for a while, but for now let's get back down to earth and the nitty-gritty of daily life.

Inner World vs Outer World

In simple terms, our daily experience is determined by our *focus*. ('Your focus determines your reality,' is the famous Jedi quote from *Star Wars: The Phantom Menace*). But most people are unaware that there is a constant flux between our inner world focus and outer world focus. 'Inner World versus Outer World sounds like a really cool space battle,' said my youngest son just now, reading over my shoulder – and, in a way, that is what it often is – a battle.

Whatever we focus on will send signals inside that trigger responses, but the receiver of those signals – our subconscious mind – seems to have a problem telling the difference between signals which come from the outer world of our senses and those which come from the inner world of our imagination.

We need to understand the difference and, more importantly, how to consciously influence and change this process if we are going to de-hypnotize ourselves and shift our behavioural patterns.

For example, if we feel nerves or anxiety when speaking in front of a group of people, as I used to, that is most likely because our inner imaginative world has conjured up an idea or vision of some sort of unpleasant outcome such as messing up and feeling stupid, rejected, embarrassed, ridiculed or inadequate. The group of people may actually be kind and keen to hear what we have to say, so the outer world in this moment is actually safe and supportive – but our inner imaginative world is busy referencing our beliefs and, in this case, creating an inner vision of a negative outcome.

This inner vision of a negative outcome triggers a fear response from our inner security system, which we experience as nerves or anxiety, and we then have to battle with this consciously while simultaneously attempting to deliver the speech.

To resolve this we either need to be able to ignore the inner imagination and switch our focus to the actual external reality, or create a more positive or beneficial inner world image for our mind to reference when faced with such a situation. But to do that consistently and effectively we also need to challenge the beliefs that triggered the fear response in the first place as very often these responses happen subconsciously, leaving us to battle something inside of us that seems out of our control.

This inner world/outer world flux is actually one of the things that sets us apart evolutionarily from other creatures and the ability to consciously reflect on the past and imagine a future is largely unique to human beings. When it works for us, it can be a great servant; when it works against us, it can be a torment and ruin our life. Many of the issues and problems we encounter in life will be owing to this inner/outer, conscious/subconscious battle, and it is all driven, once again, by our beliefs.

If we are to successfully dehypnotize ourselves from the self-imposed limitations of our life so that we can evolve, become something more and move on in some way, we must ideally do so at the level where the limitations originate.

To control symptoms, we must master the skill of switching between inner and outer world focus so that we can send the right message to our subconscious mind and we must build the psychological muscle needed to have the strength to do that. But to resolve the causes, we must also be an archaeologist of our mind to uncover the beliefs that are driving those thoughts, feelings and behaviours in the first place, beliefs which usually originate from emotive life experiences, often from so long ago that we are no longer aware of the impact they caused.

CASE STUDY: *Izzy Gets to Sleep . . . At Last!*

To illustrate the effectiveness of this inner world/outer world focus, I'd like to introduce you to someone who mastered this beautifully after a one-hour session with me. Her name is Izzy and she is eight years old. (Pay attention to the details here because it is attention to the tiny details that will enable you to tackle your own issues.)

According to her mother, Izzy had never been a good sleeper, but ever since she was six and a half her parents had noticed a more serious problem occurring at bedtimes that had been getting progressively worse over the preceding eighteen months.

'It would quite often start after she finished school,' explained Nicky, her mother. 'She would ask if she could sleep in our bed or if we could go to bed or stay upstairs when she went up. If we didn't go upstairs at her bedtime she would get really, really scared and start crying. We tried everything. We stayed upstairs with her to reassure her, but she still wouldn't go to sleep, fearing we would go downstairs. Sometimes it would be past midnight before she finally calmed down and fell asleep from exhaustion.'

Like many parents in this situation, Izzy's parents would end up cross because they felt so helpless and didn't know what to do. They would then feel guilty for being cross in this way when she was clearly so frightened, but they just couldn't see a way forward. Increasingly, they too became tired and exhausted and slowly felt less and less able to cope, until eventually it was all just too much.

'It was the most unbelievably stressful time of Izzy's life, as it was of ours,' says Nicky. 'It was affecting all of our everyday lives as, for all of us and poor Izzy, the second half of the day was filled with dread.'

Finally, in desperation, they began to look for other options and happened to come across my website and the fact that I offered to treat children.

For Izzy to have been exhibiting these kinds of extreme symptoms, I knew that she must have been believing something pretty scary and then reinforcing it with her imagination. I knew that if I could understand what this was and get her to verbalize it in a way that she never had before, there was a good chance of helping her believe and imagine something else.

I could have just dived in and gone for a positive outcome right away . . . but I also knew from experience that the closer I could get to understanding any causative ideas, the better able I would be to help create a more lasting positive outcome – otherwise we may still be trying to run up that down escalator.

After some preamble to build rapport and get Izzy opening up, I asked her to explain what it was like for her at bedtime.

'Scary,' she said.

'In what way?' I asked.

'I'm scared,' she replied.

The temptation can be to immediately try to make everything all right with reassuring words but, from experience, reassuring words that make sense to the conscious intellectual mind may not hold much weight with the more emotive, subconscious mind.

'What are you scared of?' I enquired, and she hesitated. 'What are you afraid of?' I persisted.

'Being murdered!' she suddenly revealed. 'Or taken away.'

'Being murdered or taken away?' I repeated back to her. 'By whom?'

'People breaking into my room.'

'What kind of people?'

'Bad people.'

'What kind of bad people?'

'Kidnappers,' she whispered.

'Ah, I see!' I exclaimed. 'Now I get it. You've been thinking that bad people, like kidnappers, will break into your room at night and either murder you or take you away from your mum and dad, is that right?'

She nodded.

'And every time you've been thinking that, it has been making you scared in case it really happens, is that right?'

She nodded again.

'And that's why you've been getting upset and want your mum and dad to stay with you, just in case, is that right?'

Another nod.

'Well, I don't think I would want to go to bed either if I thought that was going to happen,' I said, looking to further build rapport. 'And we're not really designed to fall asleep anyway if we feel scared, why would we? We'd need to stay awake to protect ourselves, wouldn't we?'

She nodded enthusiastically and I could see that I had her complete, undivided attention at this moment.

People may be horrified at me saying such things to a child, but actually I am just bringing into the open and repeating what has already been going through her mind. Verbalizing the inner thoughts brings the subconscious and invisible into our awareness, making them conscious and visible and therefore easier to deal with.

And there is also something powerful about having someone else verbalize back to us the exact thoughts that we have been holding inside. It forms a connection, an understanding, and builds a bridge.

I often explain it by saying that for two people to have an effective communication, they must first each lower their drawbridge, otherwise their words will probably hit a raised barrier and fall into the moat. I have watched many parents do this – and, regrettably, done exactly the same with my own children on numerous occasions, especially during my early parenting years. But when we can lower our drawbridge and enable another to feel safe enough to lower theirs, then we can have a more meaningful exchange.

As Izzy stared at me intently, I could see that her drawbridge was now fully lowered . . . but there was still a piece of the puzzle missing: Why? Why should she believe this could happen? So I asked her, using an indirect question.

'I wonder what made you believe this could happen?' I enquired casually, almost as if I was musing to myself, but I caught her gaze poignantly at the last moment.

'I don't know,' she said, looking away slightly.

As any interrogator will tell you, we cannot allow 'I don't knows', because 'I don't know' can become a learned response that allows the interviewee to avoid providing any information.

So when Izzy said, 'I don't know,' I needed to persist and dig deeper.

'Yes, that's OK,' I reassured. 'But I wonder what you imagine it might be?'

It seemed like an eternity before she answered, but she suddenly broke the silence with, 'I probably heard something on TV a long time ago.'

And now I knew what to do. What I am essentially looking for during any initial chat with any client are answers to the following:

1. What is the client actually imagining that is causing them to have a problem?
2. What clues are there as to why he or she might be thinking and believing that in the first place?

With Izzy, I was fortunate enough to find an indication of both in the first twenty minutes of this first session and we now had a plausible explanation as to what had been going through her mind.

It appeared that it may have all started some years before when she overheard something on TV about the idea of kidnappers – bad people who can break into her bedroom at night and either murder her (these are her exact words) or steal her away so that she would never see her parents again. The tragic Maddie McCann story came to mind, but I did not mention this, nor did I really need to know. But if a young child had seen such a news report and grasped the implications, such a moment would have all the elements required for implanting an idea by natural hypnosis – an increase in attention around one idea, a lack of critical analysis to reject the idea and heightened emotion, in this case, fear – to make a lasting impression that her mind would then use as a reference for future situations.

As young children, we do not have much of a reality filter, so every night Izzy had probably been going to bed feeling that it was highly likely someone would break into her home and either murder her or kidnap her. But she couldn't verbalize it in that way because it was all happening just below her usual awareness – and no one had known how to pull that information out for examination because it is not included in the parents' handbook we never receive!

I could have just calmly and rationally explained the obvious to her . . . but, again, that would be addressing the conscious, intellectual mind. I needed to bring about a change at the causative level, the place where the beliefs and imagination were firing from.

Now, with Izzy sitting in the chair a few feet in front of me, I asked her if she would be happy to play a little imagination game, 'to help her feel better at bedtime'.

'We'll get your mum to join in as well,' I said. 'That OK?'

She nodded and smiled.

I had them both close their eyes and gently guided them into what I call the 'access state' by asking them to focus on their breathing and various muscles of their body, plus a little trick I will teach you later which encourages a more inner focus.

I then had Izzy imagine she was about to go on an adventure – but not by herself. She would be accompanied by Chad and Vy – Spy Ninja characters, who I had learned earlier she was fond of – and I saw her smile at the mention.

'I want you to travel back in time,' I explained. 'Chad and Vy are with you and I want you to find that little you, the one who has just heard something scary on the TV. I want you and Chad and Vy to go up to that little you and let her know that you have come to help and that she does not need to feel on her own any more. And I want you to gather up that scary feeling inside and just blow it all away like this.'

I took some deep breaths myself and blew out noisily so that she could hear and copy.

I knew she was never actually alone at bedtime with her parents around, but the fear of that is part of the problem, so having someone there in her imagination would begin to build a new inner world for her. The blowing-out technique is something I learned many years ago from a hypnotherapy trainer called Neil French. The method involves having a child imagine travelling back through time, taking a hero figure with them for support and encouragement, and seeking out younger versions of themselves who are experiencing strong emotions. We ask the child, supported by their hero figure, to go up to the younger version of themselves and help them blow away whatever it is they are feeling. It is a great way of helping young children deal with past upsets without actually having to talk about them out loud.

We did these breaths a few times and then I said, 'I wonder how different it would feel at bedtime having Chad and Vy around to protect you and take care of the kidnappers?'

I waited for the response while she was busily testing this out in her imagination.

'Better,' she finally replied.

'Better?' I repeated. 'That's good. In what way?'

'Better,' she said again.

I thought we had made progress, but also felt we could do more because there was a specific word I was waiting for her to say.

'I wonder what it would be like if the kidnappers never got

anywhere near your bedroom in the first place?' I asked, attempting to put some distance between her and the source of the fear. 'What if Chad and Vy went out to take care of them miles away from here? I wonder what that would be like?'

There was another pause while her imagination went to work and then, 'Good,' she said.

'What would Chad and Vy actually do when they find the kidnappers?' I asked, expecting her to say 'ninja them' or something similar.

But she paused for a moment, eyes still closed, before stating, 'They would tell them to not be so stupid and silly.'

'And what would the kidnappers do then?' I asked, smiling inwardly, surprised at the wisdom of the response compared to my own more aggressive inner assumption, and also because I wanted to make sure we left no loose ends.

'They would stop and go and do something better instead,' she said, very matter-of-factly, as if I had asked a stupid question.

'And what would that be like for you, at bedtime now, knowing that Chad and Vy had done that, and the kidnapers weren't going to do that any more and were going to do something else better instead?' (I used as many of her words as possible.)

'Better,' she said again.

'In what way?' I persisted.

And then, after a long pause, 'Safe,' she finally sighed.

Bingo!

That was the word I was waiting for. *Safe.*

In order to go to sleep easily and peacefully, like all of us, she needed to feel safe. But I wanted it to come from her, not me. And now Izzy had managed to create that for herself using her own imagination, with characters and ideas that meant something to her.

With her eyes still closed, I spent a few minutes summarizing everything we had spoken about in order to help reinforce it, and added that she would be able to think of this at bedtime, and then gently asked them both to open their eyes.

That first night, Nicky put Izzy to bed at 8 p.m. as usual and she was asleep within ten minutes, whereas she had previously been awake as late as midnight!

A week or so later, Nicky sent me a note explaining that Izzy's life had been transformed as she was no longer petrified of the nights, and was happy to go to sleep by herself, a huge relief for all concerned.

Izzy had mastered her inner world so that her imagination now served her instead of enslaving her. She had updated her belief system so that she now felt safe at bedtime. And although I gave a little nudge and some guidance here and there, the key point to remember is that the actual solution came from Izzy herself. Eighteen months of fear and upset, transformed in minutes once we knew what was really going on and could address it at the right level.

The same phenomenon at play in Izzy is also happening within every one of us. Sometimes it is easy to resolve, sometimes it is a little more involved. But it is always simple – there is something we are believing that is causing us to think and feel certain things, which then affects how we behave. When we can update or transform that, our life transforms and updates accordingly.

Conscious Intellect vs Subconscious Emotion

A large part of the problem when we are seeking to resolve the issues in our lives is that we are often doing so from the perspective of our conscious, logical, intellectual mind, not our subconscious, emotional-response-level mind. This can leave us with an intellectual understanding of what we think the issue is . . . but if we still have the issue, there must be something else going on making it happen, so we need to dig deeper.

In the positive thinking, personal development and motivational world, we are often told to 'sharpen the axe', just keep going, work harder, stay positive, push, push, push, more, more, more, and of course there are times when that is useful and helps us to achieve incredible results. But no matter how many hours we spend sharpening our axe or applying our will and determination, we are never going to find gold if we are digging in the wrong place or only ever scraping the surface. We need to hit the right spot and dig there – sometimes deep, sometimes very deep – to make sure we are dealing with the real source of the issue, not just the effect.

The more easily we can get to the real root of our issues and develop a more useful mindset at that level, the less we have to do or deal with on the surface.

To do this we need the right tool and, fortunately, that tool is readily available to each one of us in the form of a naturally occurring state of mind that we are all inherently experts at already. The challenge, however, is to master it consciously, rather than have it happen subconsciously. Otherwise we spend much of our time attempting to deal with the fallout.

Natural Hypnosis: The Access State

Hypnosis is one of those words that means so many different things to different people. To me, having carried out many thousands of client sessions using hypnosis, it is just a very naturally occurring state of mind which we each drift into and out of hundreds or thousands of times a day.

Thinking back, I suspect I spent the majority of my schooldays in this state, gazing out of the window or staring at the blackboard, aware of my surroundings if need be and yet somehow unaware, my mind day-dreaming of things I would much rather have been doing. Many people also experience the same phenomenon while driving or doing any repetitive task.

We do not go 'under' hypnosis, knocked unconscious like a patient under anaesthetic – we constantly transition into it and out of it throughout our day, shifting our awareness from the outer world of our senses to the inner world of our imagination and back again, as effortlessly as we breathe.

We can drift into it slowly, as we gradually let go of the stresses and strains of life for a while, or we can jump there in an instant if something grabs our attention and causes us to focus in the right way. We do not need to meditate with incense for hours until we achieve a deep enough relaxation, nor do we even need our eyes closed – it is a state of mind, not a state of body.

Hypnosis is so normal that until we can recognize the signs, most of us do not even realize we are in it. There is nothing mystical or magical about it and we can all do it. Yet we should not be fooled by its ease and simplicity. Like electricity, although we cannot see it, we can observe the effects of it – and it is one of the most powerful and profound influencers of our lives, from the moment we are born until the moment we die.

Every time we allow ourselves to suspend critical thinking for a while, letting an idea go unchallenged, we are drifting into hypnosis. If we can suspend that critical thinking sufficiently, we may be able to use that to our benefit and introduce new ideas into the working of our mind, which can then serve us in some way. We may also be able to do the opposite, and use it to slide through the layers of memories and beliefs, accessing unresolved wounds and traumas from our past that have already made their way in, so that they can be healed, released and set free without the need for long and drawn-out therapy.

Hypnosis has nothing to do with control or being controlled, and instead is much more about a focusing of attention in a certain way. It can be induced at will, either by oneself or with the help of another, but it can also occur spontaneously whenever something in life sets up the right conditions for us, and this is what I refer to as 'natural hypnosis', though they are really one and the same.

Natural hypnosis can occur every time we focus on an idea, unchallenged – good or bad – sufficiently for it to reach our subconscious, which also includes all the self-talk we indulge in as we go through our day. If we allow the ideas and focus to persist, they get reinforced, and we may then experience the effect in our thoughts, feelings and behaviour later on down the line.

It is the process of natural hypnosis that has caused us to develop many, if not all, of our issues in the first place. Once we understand this and recognize it, we can then use the very same natural process to access and undo old ideas that have already been instilled in us by life, and instead focus on new, more positive ideas that we wish to instil in their place, bringing about deep and powerful transformations.

Because of the many connotations associated with the word 'hypnosis', however, I often avoid using that label; however much I explain, many people are still often waiting to 'get there' and be 'hypnotized' – not realizing life has already got them there!

Instead, I will use more everyday words: 'let your mind go inward for a while', 'just focus on that thought for a moment', 'stay with that feeling, and see where it takes you'.

In my own mind, I think of it as the 'access state', meaning the state of mind where we can more easily access the thoughts, feelings, memories and beliefs responsible for our issues, opening a doorway to our subconscious to release old ideas that no longer serve us, allowing new and more beneficial perspectives to arise in their place.

Hypnosis – natural hypnosis – the access state – whatever we wish to call it – allows us to drop down a level in our mind. It allows us to step back from the daily fight and gain access to the inner thoughts, feelings and emotions responsible for creating the surface-level symptoms that we experience as problems. And it allows us to reinforce or boost the positive ideas we already hold as well, so that even a brief dip into it can leave us feeling revitalized and renewed, with a fresh perspective.

Our will, focus, persistence and determination applied in this way can then be amplified dramatically.

We have seen how this process of natural hypnosis set up ideas in a child's mind, and how I was able to help reverse it and introduce new ideas that enabled her to get to sleep at last. Now let's look at how this can work for an adult by introducing you to Kate, who had become locked into a cycle of destructive relationships, conditioned through natural hypnosis, and how I used the same process to help undo this, helping her to create a more positive set of ideas to take away and integrate into life.

Again, pay attention to the details of this story because it is a good example of the various levels you may need to access in yourselves, using the exercises later, if you wish to bring about transformation in any area of your own life.

CASE STUDY: *Kate Finds the Courage to be Herself*

When Kate first contacted me for help she explained that, while she had done a lot of work on herself over the years, now aged forty-three, she had developed a pattern of attracting partners who were either incredibly controlling, toxic and judgemental or who weren't really interested in her and made her feel very unimportant to them.

Kate had an MSc in Counselling and had recently enrolled at my own Practitioner Academy, and she said, 'I realized because of my studies over the years that I was attracting these partners for some subconscious reason and therefore it was my responsibility to work out why, for any change to happen.'

I was impressed by Kate's willingness to take responsibility for her part in her recovery process, very different to those who come along saying 'fix me' or blaming everyone and everything for their woes. I never expect anyone to take responsibility for what has happened to them, but I do expect them to take responsibility for their recovery. Otherwise, they will be forever the victim.

As we started chatting through Kate's history, it became clear to me within minutes that this was a strong person, someone who had dealt with a lot in life, raised a son by herself, worked hard to overcome her past and better herself, and yet was still trapped by her own demons, which were keeping her locked in these repeating cycles of destructive relationships.

Early in the discussion, when I asked, 'So where do you think all this comes from?', she straight away told me that she had been sexually abused by a friend of her babysitter, who had just appeared one night when she was only eight years old.

'Thankfully,' she said, 'this was a one-off event,' but added that she had always been very close to her father, had had a pretty toxic relationship with her mother and that neither parent had been particularly emotionally supportive, though with hindsight she realized now this was unintended.

(As you will see, there was no coincidence in the fact that she mentioned the abuse and lack of support in the same sentence -- it is connected statements like this that will provide the clues to identifying our own invisible beliefs when we do the exercises later on.)

When Kate's parents eventually separated, Kate stayed with her mum, and from the age of twelve when her mum remarried, had a stepfather who was aggressive and abusive, verbally and mentally.

Describing these times, Kate said, 'I was a very sad child and teenager, and wouldn't wish to relive any of my childhood. I was very angry from the trauma but also because I was so suppressed as a child/teen. I wasn't ever allowed to speak out, although I did, which didn't go down well! I was labelled the "black sheep" of the family and controlled to within an inch of my life. My nails were horrendously bitten and I started to develop an eating disorder but thankfully managed to sort out the latter myself quite quickly.'

At twenty-two, while at uni, she sought counselling to assist with insomnia that had developed, but although she found the counsellor to be lovely, the advice she received was ineffectual.

From the age of twenty-seven to twenty-nine she was with a very supportive partner who loved her unconditionally, but she couldn't handle that because she felt that she didn't deserve him. She would express a lot of verbal anger towards him, usually when alcohol was involved, which she then would feel hugely guilty about afterwards.

By the time she was thirty years old, she realized she had a problem with the abuse trauma as she was experiencing severe and overwhelming insomnia along with feeling angry, anxious and fearful too.

She began to feel terrified about everyday situations and continued to use alcohol to make herself feel better.

Determined to do something about her behaviour during the recent relationship, as well as the continued insomnia, Kate sought more help, but in the end the counselling and pure relaxation hypnotherapy didn't work for her. Sad, desperate and frustrated, Kate eventually broke off the relationship with her fiancé, not because she wanted to, as she still loved him, but because she feared it was close to sending her over the edge.

Then things began to change. Throughout her thirties she worked with a different hypnotherapist on trauma release and the issues created by the relationship with her stepdad and mum. She experienced regression therapy, working with emotion around the trauma to actually release and resolve issues rather than just talking about them as the previous therapies had. In doing so, she was finally able to let go of some of the terror she used to feel around everyday situations, such as sleeping in a house on her own.

Although Kate's insomnia and general anxiety had finally begun to improve, they hadn't gone completely, and so it was a few years later, driven by yet another destructive relationship cycle, that she finally booked her first session with me.

As I sat listening to Kate's words and the way she described her situations, the patterns were immediately obvious and I suspected that no amount of coaching or counselling would ever truly resolve this. Despite her initial comments to me that she had dealt with the past and just wanted to sort out this relationship situation, I felt that, in this case, we needed to dig deeper still because these cycles don't just happen by themselves; there is always a reason and often the best way to resolve them is to dive in and go for the core.

In my early years of practice I used to think I had to be quite clever, with an array of wonderful therapeutic tools at my disposal. But with time I have come to realize that any cleverness on my part pales into insignificance compared to enabling the inner workings of someone's mind to do the work for them, from the inside. I now understand I do not need to be clever to help someone solve a lifelong issue – I just need to set the process going and help keep things on track. Most importantly, I need to make sure the client doesn't duck out of the tricky bits, the areas that in self-help usually cause us to put the book down or skip that section, or in conventional therapy try to avoid discussing.

I have learned that if you follow the feelings they will take you to the beliefs, but this is not an intellectual process – it has to be an experiential one in order to get the full release. I could see that Kate's previous hypnotherapy had done a lot of good in this direction, but experience has taught me that there are many layers and often we have to dig extra deep to get that final resolution.

As I helped Kate relax her mind and go inward, I asked her to focus on the feelings she had been experiencing and follow them, deeper inside.

What we found was a lot of unexpressed anger and also feelings of abandonment and lack of support.

(Think back to what she said at the beginning about abuse and lack of support – without knowing, she was telling me there was a link between the two and where the real issue lay that we had to get to.)

'Stay with the feelings,' I told her, 'just stay with them.' People often express a lot of anger during these kind of sessions and that is perfectly valid but I always remind them, 'Anger is a response. I wonder what the feeling or upset is underneath the anger? Feel around for the hurt, the pain, whatever it may be. Feel around for that.'

As I said this to Kate, I noticed her facial expression change as she accessed a deeper level and suddenly there was an intense welling-up. 'Why is no one there to support me when the abuse is happening? And why is there no one there afterwards?' she sobbed. 'Why?'

Kate wasn't just thinking or talking about what had happened, she was now re-experiencing the actual original feelings (in this case of abandonment and lack of support) as if she was there. This is what we call an abreaction – a reliving of the original emotive content that had been held in for all these years.

As her adult mind verbalized the childhood thoughts and as the emotional pain poured out of her, I could see this was coming from very deep inside, a purging of hurt and pain she had carried with her for thirty-five years and had been subconsciously recreating in relationship after relationship.

As the initial wave of emotions subsided, Kate's mind continued to link and connect and peel away further layers. Suddenly, the mood changed, and I saw her face change too as she shifted to a different level. Guilt.

Another wave of emotion ensued as Kate was suddenly feeling a huge amount of guilt for how she had treated people over the years, especially her fiancé, but as the previous emotions began to ease, so did the guilt.

She realized that it wasn't purely her fault. In a way, life had programmed her – 'hypnotized' her – to feel and behave that way and she was coping the best she could at the time.

I took her through an interactive visualization exercise so that she could say sorry, not just mentally, but actually verbalizing and speaking aloud, as if she was really there, which is always more effective.

With the release of the pent-up emotions and an easing of the guilt, a new level of insight flooded in. Kate realized she had been feeling and believing that 'men couldn't be trusted' and she was 'supposed to feel abandoned and unsupported' – that's how life had hypnotized her – causing her to repeatedly seek out relationships that fulfilled those ideas and to reject ones that didn't.

But as the veil lifted, she now understood that she didn't need to do that any more.

Kate went on a journey to the emotional core of her problems and released the emotionally charged beliefs she had been carrying with her for all these years. This then allowed the space for new ideas to form. I rarely need to introduce ideas of my own to help and support the client. What happens is, as we fully experience the old idea and the emotion around it, it dissolves away by itself and, sometimes aided by a few pertinent questions, a new more positive idea begins to grow in its place, which we can then reinforce. My job is simply to give a little nudge of encouragement and to help the client become aware of the new ideas forming to speed up the process.

Towards the end of a session, I will always encourage the client to find some kind of 'I can' summary statement that they can take away with them, to help them assimilate what has happened and move on in life.

With Kate it was 'I can begin to trust the right kind of men now'. We didn't want her openly trusting everybody because that would leave her vulnerable to more abuse and, conversely, we didn't want her not trusting anybody, because that would mean she would never allow herself to be open to a loving relationship. So we needed her mind to be more discerning.

This whole session lasted just over an hour and, a few months afterwards, Kate told me that although she had still attracted a couple of people who weren't going to be very good for her and almost dated them, she could now see the red flags a lot quicker and more clearly and dodged the bullet, so to speak!

She said the session made her much more aware of what she should and shouldn't put up with. Her self-esteem and self-worth were a lot higher and she was learning that she was actually a good person.

Things continued to improve for Kate, but she contacted me six months later for some more help. She had been friends with someone for nearly a year but hadn't ever considered him as any more than a friend, partly because she thought she would let him down in some way and 'wouldn't be good enough for him'.

'The barriers were well and truly up,' said Kate, 'and whatever he said, I wasn't open to hearing it! The signs were all there that he was a loving, caring, kind, patient man but the only thing I could hear was me screaming "NOOOOOOOOO!" in my head to any suggestion of us being a couple!'

This 'not being good enough' was the feeling hook I was looking for so, again, I helped Kate relax and go inward, following the feeling to wherever it would take us, in search of emotionally charged ideas or beliefs. We found the answer amongst all the details we had previously talked about, but an idea she had not yet fully verbalized or brought into conscious awareness.

I see this so often. It's not that people are unaware that what they have been through has caused them problems, but more that they are unaware of the full emotional impact it has had on them. Very often we may revisit scenes or ideas that clients have spent years discussing in therapy, with them assuring me they are over it, and yet there, very often shielded by layers of protection, are the unexpressed thoughts, feelings and emotions that have been causing all their problems. A different client said to me quite recently, after a particularly transformative session, 'I thought we were looking for something I had repressed or forgotten about, but the answer was there, hiding in plain sight all along.' That's why I think the phrase 'invisible beliefs' is very apt.

As we dug into this 'not being good enough' idea with Kate, we had an even deeper release than before, and I knew we had got somewhere profound; this wasn't just about self-worth or self-esteem, this was about her ultimate validity and right to exist as a person. In answer to the question uncovered in our previous session, 'Why was no one there to support me?', the answer her mind came up with was, 'Because I am not worth supporting . . . and if even my parents don't want to support me then why would anyone else? It must be me. I am just not good enough.'

Again, this was no calm, rational discussion, this was an incredibly intense release of raw emotion, with Kate sobbing uncontrollably as the lifetime of suppressed and repressed emotions came flooding out – 'I am simply not good enough as a person.'

This was the emotive response I was looking for in this type of session. I felt we had reached the bottom of the pit, so to speak, and therefore decided it was time to help put Kate back together. If we left it at this point, there would still be the benefit of having accessed the core emotion, but at these moments we tend to be very open and so it is a great time to introduce more positive and beneficial ideas in order to speed up the healing process.

I could have just offered some ideas myself but I always prefer them to come from the client, if possible, so I said, 'I wonder if the adult you, the one sat here talking with me, could go back in time now and be with that little you, the one who was feeling so

49

unsupported. I wonder if you could walk up to her, look into her little eyes and let her know who you are. And that you have come to help. So that she doesn't haven't to feel on her own any more.'

More tears flowed for Kate but this time they were 'happy' tears.

'What's that like,' I enquired, wanting her to verbalize but also not wishing to interrupt the moment, 'having someone be there for you?'

I was deliberately vague, so that she now didn't know whether to be the adult or the child, and her mind was most likely switching back and forth between the two. But she just nodded and smiled, and I could see that she was now experiencing what it felt like to be supported.

As the tears flowed more gently and the emotions subsided, I could see that she was coming back as someone new. She had released the old belief that was causing her so much unhappiness and begun to develop a new, more positive one, of feeling worthy of support and therefore worthy of love and all that goes with it.

'I can let him love me now,' she said quietly as we gently brought the session to a close. I asked her to repeat it, numerous times, and she smiled. 'I can let him love me now.'

Speaking about the experience some weeks later, Kate explained, 'It literally felt like a switch had gone off in my head and body and I was allowing myself to realize that I was a good person, that some-one kind could love me, that I deserved that and that I wasn't going to let them down.

'I didn't need to put up all the "yeah but" protection barriers. I could live in the present more too, but most importantly I could also just be myself, which I'm not sure I've ever really been "allowed" to be, and, wow, does that make me a happier person!'

By being brave enough to follow the feelings, Kate had truly faced her past, herself and her fears, and evolved beyond measure. She had dehypnotized herself from her previous beliefs and found something more real underneath. She went on to have a loving and meaningful relationship with the new friend, her family relation-ships resolved as well, and she now uses the wisdom and insight gained in order to help others who have been in similar situations.

Creating the Right Conditions

For many of us there will be an inner conflict that has been making it difficult for us to create the right conditions to achieve whatever it is we wish to achieve. Only when we resolve that inner conflict will we be able to move on more easily and effortlessly. That conflict is usually created by an invisible belief. Think back to the examples so far:

Izzy – Before
My parents want me to be able to go to sleep by myself
[conflicts with]
I cannot go to sleep by myself because I am petrified
    (because I do not feel safe)
[invisible belief creates stress]

It is a stalemate until we can dissolve one or more of the underlying beliefs, which then resolves the conflict and thus allows us to create the right conditions.

Izzy – After
My parents want me to be able to go to sleep by myself
I can go to sleep by myself now because I am safe
We are all happy

We had to go on an adventure into Izzy's memories, beliefs and imagination to resolve that conflict, so that her feeling safe could feel true. But once the conflict was resolved, Izzy evolved to become a person who can now go to sleep by herself at bedtime, and everyone is happy.
Now think about Kate.

Kate – Before
I want a loving relationship
[conflicts with]
I don't trust men and don't deserve to be loved
[invisible belief creates anxiety and unhappiness]

We cannot have both ideas existing side by side because it just doesn't work and creates stress, tension, anxiety and a whole host of symptoms and adaptive behaviours.

However, when we delved into her thoughts, actions, memories, feelings and emotions, challenged any beliefs and assumptions behind these statements and dissolved any emotions that were supporting them, suddenly we could have a resolution.

Kate – After

I want a loving relationship

I can trust the right kind of man and feel worthy of love and
respect

I can have a happy loving relationship now

So as we are examining our thoughts, feelings and emotions, we need to identify any conflicts between what we consciously desire and subconsciously feel and believe. And once we can resolve that conflict, the new idea naturally comes into being – we don't necessarily need to affirm it a thousand times a day, though a little nudge can be helpful.

Feeling Rather Than Thinking

While Kate is a remarkable person for facing up to what she has been through, and the results themselves may seem remarkable compared to longer, more conventional therapies, these are quite usual when working in this way because 'feeling rather than thinking' usually helps us get to the core of an issue more quickly and more easily.

We could have spent a long time talking and putting strategies in place to deal with the various surface-level symptoms, but in this case they would all have been attempts to run up that down escalator. By following the feelings, and working at that level, we were able to flip the switch and bring about a much deeper release. *Then* the positive ideas and strategies can have much greater impact, resulting in an overall deeper and lasting transformation.

Questions, then, might be: *How can we do this for ourselves? Can we, even? Or are we obliged to see a therapist if we want to escape the limitations of our life and finally become that something more? Do we always need to go back to the past? Or are there other ways? Shouldn't we just become more mindful or set goals and do relentless positive affirmations until we get there?*

From my experience, although it is often easier and faster to have someone take us through such exercises, the answer is yes, we can do this for ourselves, provided we are willing to face what we are really feeling and follow where it takes us.

I would also say that we do not necessarily need to dig around in our past every time looking for causes, though it can sometimes be extremely beneficial to do so. And positive thinking, affirmations and mindfulness can be powerful tools for change when used in the right way – but it depends on the specific issues or areas we are seeking to change, and how we use them, as I will explain shortly.

For now, let's dig a little deeper into the understanding of how we end up feeling the way we feel and behaving the way we do, so that we have an even better understanding of which approach will work best for us when seeking to make any changes.

Something that I believe is absolutely vital in all of this is a process known as the 'threat response', which affects virtually every thought, feeling, action and decision we make, consciously and subconsciously, throughout our day, and is very often the means by which natural hypnosis occurs in the first place.

The Threat Response

When our mind perceives any kind of 'threat', an automatic animal sur-vival system kicks in. This system, also referred to as the 'stress response', 'alarm response' or 'fight or flight "F" response', is designed for short-term activation to help us deal with immediate threat or danger.

It automatically prepares us to physically engage an aggressor (fight) while planning for injury and repair afterwards, or to withdraw and run away (flight), or both. It can cause us to become immobile (freeze) in the hope that 'it' – the aggressor – won't see us. It can also cause us to become subordinate (fawn), like dogs rolling over, and in extreme cases it can even cause us to collapse (feign/feint), like an animal playing dead, until the threat has passed.

The whole process works by our senses first sending information to a part of the brain called the amygdala. If the amygdala perceives evi-dence of danger or threat, it rapidly sends an alarm signal to another part of the brain called the hypothalamus, which then communicates with the rest of the body through the autonomic nervous system, made up of two components:

1. Sympathetic nervous system – the main function of which is to activate a biological cascade of physiological changes to prepare the body to deal with the threat.
2. Parasympathetic nervous system – the main role of which is to put the brakes on and return the body to its normal resting state once the threat has passed.

This biological cascade largely consists of the release of two hormones, adrenaline and cortisol.

Adrenaline increases our heart rate (aided by the vagus nerve releas-ing the brakes), increases our blood pressure and triggers a boost in our energy supplies. Cortisol (also known as the 'stress hormone') causes an increase in glucose (for energy) in the bloodstream, ramps up our brain's ability to use that glucose and increases the availability of substances that repair tissues.

Cortisol also reduces or shuts down any systems that would be non-essential or detrimental to a dangerous fight or flight situation. This may include suppressing the digestive system (hence anxiety can cause loss of appetite), suppressing the reproductive system (hence stress can cause sexual issues, including loss of libido) and suppressing the growth processes. In other words, when under attack, 'Divert all non-essential power to the weapons and shields.'

All of this is a wonderful mechanism that greatly enhances our chances of survival in a dangerous situation. The problem is, our minds can trigger the same response – or some of it, at least – towards a *psychological* threat, real or imagined, in exactly the same way as if there were a physical threat present.

In its simplest of forms, anger, anxiety and procrastination, for example, are displays of fight, flight or freeze, respectively. Being good, always trying to appease or avoiding conflict are displays of fawn.

But it can be less obvious as well. If we feel we are lacking, in any way, the threat response can activate the desire to go out there and get 'it', whatever 'it' may be, in order to appease the sense of lack. Lack of money, lack of love, lack of self-worth and lack of security are all powerful drivers that may trigger behaviours in us designed to compensate or rectify the situation. Make money, find love, gain a sense of worth, make ourselves safe, for example. Sometimes these compensating and adaptive behaviours can be incredibly useful. Other times they can be utterly destructive. Or a mixture of the two, which can be confusing.

The 'threat' does not always need to be actually happening now, in the present, however. We can have a threat response in the present to something that we *imagine* may happen in the future – even if we are completely safe right now. Or we can have a threat response to something that has already happened in the past and is over and done with, yet causes us suffering when we remember it. Our *imagination* can activate the threat response by bringing something to mind, creating the very same physical and biological symptoms as if it were happening now.

These responses to threat – whether physical or psychological, real or imagined, past, present or future – along with the adaptive

measures and outcomes they generate, are what create many – if not
all – of our surface-level symptoms.

It is these responses we are usually looking to change whenever we
seek help in some way, whether through interaction with another or in
the form of self-help.

It is important to acknowledge, however, that this threat response is
an automatic, subconscious process, and activates faster than we can consciously think. While our conscious mind may take 500ms (half a second)
to work out we are in danger and begin a response, our subconscious
will usually have activated within just 12ms (that's forty times faster) – or
5ms (a hundred times faster) in the case of a loud noise, which is why we
instinctively jump when startled by loud sounds.

Because the automatic, subconscious threat response works faster
than we can consciously think, our fear or anxiety often gets activated
before we have had a chance to think logically and rationally about a
situation.

**It can then feel as if we are divided and left battling something
inside of us, but outside of our control, as the something inside takes
over.**

The result is we then not only have to deal with the situation
itself – speaking in public, walking up to someone to introduce ourselves
or completing a piece of work on time – but also have to simultaneously
deal with our inner threat response, which may be yelling 'Get me out
of here!'

To further complicate things, as soon as the threat response kicks in,
it tries to reduce rational thinking by directing blood flow away from the
logic centres at the front of the brain and into the amygdala, the emotional response area at the centre. The message is very simple: 'Don't
sit around thinking about what to do, either fight or get away.' This can
cause us to behave in ways that seem very irrational at times, until the
perceived threat has passed, whereupon we return to 'normal', often
wondering what just happened.

**Learning to reduce, manage or eliminate the threat response is
therefore a vital component of any personal transformation process.**

The labelling of information we are receiving from our senses – or
imagination – as being a potential threat will be coming from the beliefs

we hold about the incoming information, however, *not* the information or situation itself.

The thought of sitting an exam can be a very natural, enjoyable process to someone who feels confident in their knowledge and keen to express it in order to gain some kind of certification and move on with life. But the same situation to someone else may mean the possibility of failure, disappointment, of letting people down, a life ruined, and so create fear, stress and anxiety. This is why understanding our *response* to a situation is important, not necessarily the situation itself.

Our response to a situation – whether a real or imagined situation, past, present or future – will give us an indication of the *beliefs* we hold – often very consciously – about a particular situation. These beliefs were created by our life experiences, now stored in our subconscious mind as memories, sustained and reinforced by repetition and focus on them.

So we can use the events in life that trigger us as *signposts*, *indicators* or *clues* as to where we need to look, and by following the feelings we can uncover our beliefs – even the invisible ones – as well as the ancient pains, traumas or events that caused them.

Any time we feel or sense any kind of threat – real or imagined, physical or psychological – our inner security system will go into alert and begin to encourage us to take adaptive measures to deal with it. What most people do is get caught up in the responses and adaptive measures. What we are going to do instead is go a level deeper, figure why the threat response was triggered in the first place and find ways to reduce or eliminate it.

But here is the sting: this threat response can also kick in when we are attempting to tackle our personal problems! It will activate, albeit sometimes very subtly, to help protect us from thinking about what we don't want to think about, or feeling what we don't want to feel, and *create further surface-level symptoms*.

Someone with an alcohol or drug problem, for example, may be choosing that as a means of self-medication to help them avoid feeling what they do not want to feel (flight). But if we try to remove their 'medication' or even try to talk about it, the threat response may kick in at this level and they may then get angry and defensive (fight), creating a second set of symptoms.

With clients, I often have to encourage them to 'stay with the feeling' for a while, to break through this, and this is something we need to learn to do ourselves if we are to break the patterns at the deepest level. When we can be brave enough to feel what we really feel – which includes the thoughts and ideas creating the threat response – we can come out the other side and no longer need to respond, react or adapt in the same way as before.

The more we are able to do this, the greater the progress we can make.

One other point to mention is that the threat response is designed to help us cope with short-term danger. It is not designed for long-term activation, and when this happens, such as during prolonged periods of stress or anxiety, the very biological processes designed to help us manage immediate threat begin to turn against us, often having an extremely detrimental effect on our physical health as well, as we shall discuss later.

Raw Emotive Content

As we go through life, our past will load us up with experiences, many of which will be quite emotional. The good ones we are usually happy to think about; the not-so-good ones less so – we may even actively try to avoid remembering them because of what they make us feel. 'I don't want to talk about it!' is a classic example.

Yet whatever impact they may have had upon us or whatever beliefs we may have developed as a result, life just keeps bringing experiences to us that reflect those beliefs . . . and with them will often come a re-experiencing of the same or similar emotion – different story, same feeling – the very same feeling or emotion we have been trying to avoid. This continues until, one day, we finally *feel* what we have been avoiding, acknowledge what we have been believing, break the pattern and move on.

And this 'feeling we have been avoiding' feeling is what I refer to as the 'raw emotive content' – the unfiltered, unedited, emotional content of a memory or experience, or the ideas and beliefs we have held on to or developed as a result of those experiences. Not the polite version we may be willing to talk about with friends or in traditional therapy – I mean the real, raw, guttural feeling that we are nearly always too scared to admit even to ourselves, let alone another.

The problem is, who wants to voluntarily feel something they most definitely do not want to feel? Who wants to feel desperation, loneliness, helplessness, entrapment, self-loathing, powerlessness, vulnerability, defencelessness, fear, shame, weakness, insignificance, guilt and worthlessness amongst many other things?

If we have a deliberate intent to do so as part of a therapeutic process perhaps, yes, we may be willing. But in everyday life, if we start to go anywhere near these feelings, we consciously and subconsciously begin to protect ourselves – we go into a reactive or adaptive mode, changing how we think, feel or behave in order to avoid it.

This avoidance of the raw emotive content, and of our beliefs, creates surface-level symptoms by influencing how we think, feel and behave, yet simultaneously helps us create more situations that are likely to bring it up. The net result is that we get caught in *Groundhog Day*-type loops – creating the opportunity to evolve and be free but being too scared to do so, thus going round the cycle again and again.

In case you were tempted to carry out a little mental bullying on yourself for not having sorted this out yet, do be aware that this avoidance of feeling is often a subconscious process, caused by the threat response. It is, however, one that we can learn to take conscious control over, which we will explore in the second part of this book.

For now, understand that beliefs, surface-level symptoms and the threat response are inextricably linked, and an understanding of this is vital for you to be able to accelerate your own personal development and freedom from limitations.

Habits, Conditioning and Hebbian Learning

While many of the emotional conditions in life we are seeking to change are caused by the threat response, we do also need to take note of the role of other factors in forming any habits or behaviours we wish to break.

My partner, Alison, runs a baking business and for a while we had large stores of ingredients at home. We didn't just have bags of flour, sugar and chocolate buttons, we had sacks of them – large ones.

I remember one day catching my son grabbing a handful of said chocolate buttons and instinctively calling out, 'Oi!', about to tell him off. Realizing this would be a little hypocritical – because I too had grabbed a handful now and then – I instead announced, 'Chocolate tax,' and held out my hand.

It took him a moment to understand, and then he dropped a few of the buttons into my hand and wandered off. The same thing happened again later and after a while he would even seek me out to pay his 'taxes' to me!

I got used to this and began to have a few chocolate buttons every time he – or I – walked into the kitchen, until eventually I couldn't walk into the kitchen without thinking of having a few chocolate buttons. I had developed a chocolate button habit, linked to my kitchen at home!

There is a phenomenon in our brain known as 'Hebbian learning', postulated by neuroscientist Donald Hebb in 1949, which is often simplified as 'neurons that fire together, wire together', although it is actually slightly more complex than that.

For our purposes here, we just need to understand that whenever we do something repeatedly, our brains form neural pathways that become more established each time we use them, like a well-trodden path through the woods. And, conversely, each time we do not use an existing pathway, our brain allows it to diminish, so that it effectively becomes overgrown and harder to navigate. Repeated use strengthens the pathways; lack of use weakens them, like muscles.

'Practice makes perfect' is a practical example of how this applies, although I prefer 'Practice makes *permanent*'* (which means we need to be careful what we practise!).

What's important to understand, though, is that repetition not only forges stronger neural pathways; if similar neural pathways fire at similar times, they can enhance each other or 'fire' together. The effect is that two separate acts such as a) walking into my kitchen and b) eating chocolate buttons can become connected or 'wired together' and their firings have a relationship – if one fires, so does the other, and this connection then becomes a well-trodden path as well. One thing triggers another and we have a conditioned response or habit.

When I do [A], I do [B].

We can apply this to virtually any repeated action in life – eating, smoking and drinking are obvious examples – but it appears that our brains also forge these pathways in relation to emotional responses so that an emotional response – including the threat response – can become a well-trodden path too. In fact, our brains get more efficient at firing any response, the more it is used.

The interesting thing is what happens when we try to change it. When I walked into my kitchen one day and discovered that the chocolate buttons had been moved (someone had – hmm – caught on), I felt as though there was 'something missing'. And this 'something missing' feeling created unease – 'something's not right' – triggering a mild form of the threat response again.

If I had allowed myself to focus on the unease, I would have had to go and find something to replace the thing I perceived to be missing (in this case, chocolate buttons), in order to feel at peace again, which is what I did at first, rummaging around the cupboards. But when I recognized what was happening and decided to sit with the feeling for a moment instead of reacting to it, I was able to address it at the causative level and thereby switch off the threat response, breaking the association and conditioning within a few days.

As the two neural pathways no longer fired together, the connecting

* I learned this phrase from Geoffrey Colvin's book *Talent is Overrated*.

path became unused, overgrown, and the association disappeared, along with the habitual behaviour.

The same is true for any habit we wish to break. If we try to just stop something or do something different, there will be a 'something's missing' element, creating the desire to get back to normal so we can relax – eat the food, go on a date, drink the wine, smoke the cigarette, beat the competitor, whatever.

> *When I do [A], I do [B].*
> *When I feel [X], I do [Y].*
> *If I don't . . . . I'll feel stressed [threat response].*

Even if the threat response may not have actually caused a habitual-type behaviour or issue in our life, we do have to be aware of it when seeking to make changes because it will otherwise make that change more difficult.

We'll go through how to do that later as well, but there is just one more thing to be aware of with this conditioning process: we mirror the people around us as we grow up.

The influential figures in our lives during our formative years and afterwards will be telling and showing us how to be. Any time we *accept* how they are and what they are teaching us – by their words or by their actions – natural hypnosis occurs and by repetition we then condition ourselves to be the same way. It becomes who we are and what we do.

> **When this happens, I am supposed to do this.**
> **When that happens, I am supposed to do that.**

But can't we just tell ourselves otherwise?

Affirmations or Lies?

If you have ever read anything remotely related to 'positive thinking', you will have come across the concept of affirmations. These are words or phrases that we are supposed to repeat to ourselves to help us change how we think, feel or behave.

I love using these with clients and on myself, though I prefer the word 'mantra', meaning 'instrument of the mind' (or that is the definition I choose to believe, anyway).

The problem is, many positive affirmations are not really doing much positive affirming and instead are actually creating an inner conflict which leads to a negative, detrimental effect instead of a positive one.

Let's use our two cases so far, Izzy and Kate, to illustrate this because you will see that the final beliefs each were able to accept are actually very good examples of affirmations or mantras.

A more direct self-help-type approach would have Izzy or Kate thinking about what they want right from the start: Izzy, to be able to go to sleep by herself (or at least that's what her parents wanted for her); and for Kate, a happy, loving relationship. They would then repeat these phrases or write them on a mirror or stick them on a fridge, or wherever, in order to be reminded of them.

I can go to sleep by myself now.
I can have a happy, loving relationship now.

This can be useful if the phrases create the right feeling or emotion. But, very often, if we jump ahead too quickly without paying attention to the underlying beliefs causing the issues, this process may actually have a detrimental effect. It may leave us feeling deflated because it 'didn't work', and we are no different to how we were before, or worse still, it may aggravate the original symptoms by creating an inner conflict – which may then fire off the threat response, leading to a host of further adaptive behaviours.

Let's look at our two examples so far:

> *Typical affirmation: I can go to sleep by myself now.*
>
> *Original inner response: No! I cannot! Because I might be murdered or kidnapped, so I am going to cry and insist my parents stay with me.*
>
> *Typical affirmation: I can have a happy and loving relationship now.*
>
> *Original inner response: No! I cannot! Because I cannot trust men and do not even deserve that, so I am going to be with men who abuse me and I will act aggressively to those who are nice.*

If we had asked Izzy or Kate to repeat these 'positive' affirmation phrases at the beginning, they would have been consciously and intellectually making those statements while subconsciously and emotionally resisting them. They would most likely have actually exacerbated the symptoms because the affirmations directly contradicted their beliefs, creating conflict, and no amount of willpower or persistence would change this.

Affirmations and mantras can be incredibly powerful when used in the right way, but for now, if we are using any kind of affirmation or mantra that actually makes us feel some kind of angst inside when we say it, *we would be better served by exploring our beliefs causing the angst*, and then creating some positive ideas around that, instead of blindly repeating the more surface-level affirmation. The same is true for any technique that involves a similar process.

This is why discerning between symptoms and causes is so important. If we create affirmations and positive mantras designed to tackle the surface-level symptoms, we may get some temporary benefit or relief, but while we are battling the zombies or lesser villains we may unwittingly be provoking the zombie master villain behind it all, whom we are, as yet, ill-equipped to deal with.

When we can understand the cause – and by that I mean the beliefs – verbalize them to help release any charged emotion and *then* create positive affirmations and mantras around that, then we can strike a powerful blow at exactly the right spot and begin to feel the change. Especially if we can use a state like natural hypnosis to enhance the process.

The problem is, while most of us are very keen to tackle the symptoms and say, 'Great, tell me what to do so I can get on with it,' we often have huge inner resistance to tackling or even acknowledging the real causes. This is another reason why self-help can be difficult and therapy can take a long time. As mentioned earlier, we are brilliant at avoiding that which we do not want to feel!

If we are to bring about real, deep, lasting transformation in any area of our life, we need to stop running from the feelings, stop trying to avoid what we don't want to feel, and instead allow ourselves to honestly acknowledge what we are really thinking and feeling, and deal with the causes of that.

Resistance is Futile

In the therapeutic environment, whenever a client is avoiding talking about an issue or facing up to something, we can say that they are 'resisting' and it can be frustrating to come up against this at first. In self-help and many talky therapies, it is very, very easy to resist – in fact, we are experts at it! But this resistance, if sustained, will actually prevent us from making the changes required to gain a deeper sense of happiness.

I remember reading that American hypnotist Gil Boyne once said, 'If you say the client is resisting, you are stealing their money,' and this always came back to me whenever I encountered what seemed to be resistance. If I was not allowed to blame the client, then there had to be something I could do! So I started experimenting with clients' resistance whenever it came up.

Instead of trying to bypass it or push to be more positive, I started following the resistance itself, and discovered that the very mechanism that seemed to keep a door locked was actually the key to unlocking it, once we fully understood how it worked and why it was there, keeping the door locked, in the first place.

Resistance is what keeps our real selves locked away. Any attempt at avoiding dealing with the resistance is therefore, ultimately, futile. We can delay but we cannot avoid because in that wonderful way that they do, life or our mind or both will find a means to keep presenting 'locked door' experiences to us that seem to be barring our path to happiness.

Our usual response of trying to bang, kick or rattle the door at first, and then seek another way through if this one remains closed, is also ultimately futile if we wish to evolve beyond these experiences. We need to realize that if we can pause and deal with the resistance itself, we can very often unlock the door, step through and never experience that type of problem ever again. Alternatively, we may actually look through that now open door and realize, 'You know what, it doesn't seem that appealing now after all,' and calmly walk away to a different, better option.

Either way, the ability to recognize resistance, follow it, understand it and resolve the ideas behind it is a key factor in unlocking our authentic, real selves and making life better.

All Resistance is Fear

Remember this: *All resistance is fear.* Saying 'I don't know' is another classic example, when we actually *do* know, but don't want to say. The areas we most want to avoid are usually the ones we most need to tackle, when approached in the right circumstances, in the right way, at the right time.

If, at this point, you are itching to get on with it, I completely understand, but we need to be sure you are not chasing the cure and unwilling to take the medicine! In Part Two, I will lead you step by step through a series of exercises designed to gently deal with all of this, but remember we may be dealing with the threat response at two levels.

The first level will be creating the original surface-level symptoms and problems, and the second level, if present, will be creating resistance to letting go of them.

All resistance is fear. But what are we fearful of? Simple. Feeling something we don't want to feel. What we must do, if we are to resolve our own issues at the deepest possible level, is go past the fear that makes us avoid feeling and instead face the real feelings and emotions we are carrying inside along with the ideas behind them.

Any time we can do that – sometimes simply by pausing long enough to acknowledge what is really going on – we immediately reduce the power of it and, in so doing, naturally begin to deprogramme or de-hypnotize ourselves, allowing more positive ideas to take their place.

This is what I did with Izzy – getting her to verbalize and express her belief about the fear of being murdered or kidnapped – and again with Kate – her fear of being so utterly worthless as a person that even her parents did not support her in her moment of need. In each case, I helped them to face up to the feelings they had been protecting themselves from feeling and go past that to find more useful and beneficial ideas instead.

I believe that transformation at the deepest level is not so much a case of 'doing something', but more a case of 'undoing something'. Allowing an old idea that we have been invisibly, subconsciously acting upon for some time – often many, many years – to finally be brought into the open for examination, so that we can feel the feeling we have been avoiding and finally be free of it to get on with life.

Any reluctance or resistance to this idea will be based on a fear and many if not all of our dysfunctional thoughts, feelings and behaviours are no more than attempts to protect ourselves from feeling what we really feel.

The very system that is supposed to help protect us from life ends up protecting us from ourselves and ultimately limiting our progress.

To me, any personal evolution will involve us facing up to anything we currently do not want to feel, so that we no longer have to carry out adaptive responses – what I have called surface-level symptoms – and instead can be more authentic.

Every time we do this, we are allowing more and more of our real selves – the Real You – to come to the surface.

The Critical Faculty, Gatekeeper of the Mind

Have you ever encountered someone for whom the answer to their problem seems so obvious to you, but no matter what you say or do, they just can't see it or accept it? Have you ever tried to tell yourself something positive, but for whatever reason it just won't go in? Have you ever noticed how some of us can more easily accept the negative things we think people are saying, but brush aside any positive remarks?

Think of it this way. Recently, my daughter and a friend were refused entry into a nightclub because my daughter was wearing tracksuit bottoms which were not allowed on that particular evening. Determined to find a way, she and her friend walked a short distance until they were out of sight of the club entrance, whereupon they fashioned a makeshift skirt from my daughter's friend's jacket! Wearing her new 'skirt', my daughter and friend headed back to the club to try their luck.

'Ah, you got changed!' said the doorman, smiling, letting them in with a friendly chat on the way.

The same person refused entry moments earlier was now allowed in, just packaged slightly differently. And this is what we must often do when seeking to introduce new, more positive ideas into our mind. Package them differently – or better still, get the door policy changed so that they are allowed in!

Whenever we attempt to introduce new ideas in order to solve a problem or bring about change and transformation, we have to get past our very own protective system – which I sometimes refer to as the 'critical faculty, gatekeeper of the mind'.

If we attempt to introduce an idea that goes *against* our existing beliefs or identity, our critical faculty may not only refuse it entry but may also trigger the threat response as a *protection* against the new idea – which we then experience as symptoms or resistance.

Many of us run up against this when following self-help advice or looking to make changes via any kind of intervention. The attempt to bring about change runs up against the critical faculty, creating resistance, barring our way, like the door security at a nightclub.

In reality we are the owner and have set the door policy which our own critical faculty now operates for us, but have become locked out of our own venue and cannot get back in. If we take on security directly, they may not recognize who we are and so they will fight back and eject us. But if we can get inside far enough to have a chat with the manager, we can regain control and set things straight.

When we are younger, we have very little, if any, critical faculty. If an authority figure tells us something, either directly using words or implied by their actions, there is no gatekeeper to check whether we should accept it or not – the idea gets in and becomes part of who we are.

Many of the fears, anxieties, doubts and limiting ideas we hold about ourselves and life are only there because they have made their way past the critical faculty – or were allowed in by it – when we were younger, because we had no reason to challenge the ideas.

'You are so stupid!'
'I am? OK, I'm stupid.'

Any time we accept an idea, unchallenged, we can say that a form of natural hypnosis has occurred, and one definition of hypnosis states that for there to be hypnosis there must be a lowering of the critical faculty.

When young, our critical faculty is barely even formed yet, so virtually any idea can enter and take root. As we develop, the critical faculty gets stronger and we become more discerning, but it's as if any ideas already in there, once inside, become part of the door policy and influence what follows, inviting in more of the same.

If, as a child, I believe 'I am stupid', anything that reflects this idea is allowed in. Anything that doesn't is not. This continues, both consciously and subconsciously, often throughout adulthood, until we begin to challenge the process.

Many people seek out hypnotherapy, asking the hypnotherapist to 'reprogramme their subconscious mind', but what they are really asking for is help to reduce or bypass their critical faculty so that more desirable ideas can be allowed in.

A good therapist or hypnotherapist can facilitate this, but it is important to realize that the change occurs from the client themselves. *All hypnosis is really self-hypnosis.*

Whoever or whatever causes us to think or feel something, which in turn makes us believe something, it is <u>our focus and acceptance of the idea, unchallenged, that creates the natural hypnosis.</u>

In some people, it is much easier to distract the critical faculty than others, and it is these people that a stage performer is looking for in their audience. These are the people who can suspend analytical thinking and focus on one idea to the exclusion of all others, so much so that the idea they focus on begins to feel real and the imagination takes over.

But for most of us in adult life, our critical faculty will be checking to see if the incoming information fits in with our current beliefs or not. And if it doesn't, we will seek to reject it, which is why we often end up back at the bottom of that escalator, feeling down and fed up because the attempt at change 'didn't work' again.

This process is at work nearly every moment of the day, as I hope you are beginning to realize, because we are constantly drifting into and out of what I call the access state, where natural hypnosis can occur, and constantly talking to ourselves. When we attempt to introduce ideas that the critical faculty, gatekeeper of the mind, does not agree with, at some level we will reject the ideas and there will be no change. But if an idea – including negative self-talk – fits our beliefs, it can walk boldly past the critical faculty unchallenged and into our subconscious, thereby affirming and reaffirming existing ideas – even if they have a negative impact on us.

Later, we will go through how to prevent this and create positive mantras that do actually work, but for now I hope you have an understanding as to why, if ever you have tried to talk positively to yourself, you may have met resistance. The critical faculty is that little voice at the back of your mind, that feeling in your body, saying, 'Who are you kidding?!'

One of the reasons I often spend a long time chatting with clients when we first meet is that I am trying to get a feel for their beliefs – the door policy of their club – so that I can get invited inside for a meeting, rather than be locked outside scuffling with security.

For now, just be aware that for the introduction of new ideas to work in this way, we may have to repackage them, like my daughter wangling her way into the nightclub. Or, better still, we can dig a little deeper and update the door policy of the club itself – our beliefs – so that the critical faculty is now happy with the new ideas.

Librarians, Monkeys and Stress

Let's just do a quick recap now to summarize everything we have covered so far, and relate it to how we can begin to make the changes we desire.

As we go through life, we receive information via our senses, and we give that information meaning, storing it as meaningful memories in our subconscious mind, like books in a vast library.

Some of those memories have very positive meanings attached, some are fairly neutral and some are very negative, with infinite shades in between. Whenever these experiences introduce ideas, which we focus on and accept, unchallenged, a process of natural hypnosis occurs, programming how we think, feel and behave from then on.

Referring to the Library Model diagram (p. 75), every time we receive more information (1) our mind scans inside, like an 'inner librarian', to find out what this new information may mean and what we can expect to happen (2), so that we have an idea what we should do. This inner librarian, however, seems to have trouble discerning between information coming from the external physical world of our senses and the internal world of our imagination.

Our librarian does not scan every single memory, every single time though – that would be a little inefficient. Instead, there is a handy reference section, which we call our beliefs. Our beliefs act like a summary of what we know so far, based on our interpretation of events and the natural hypnosis that has occurred.

If our beliefs tell our librarian that everything is OK and all clear (3a) about this new piece of incoming information, we feel calm, relaxed, normal or even good (4a). If, however, our beliefs indicate any potential for threat (3b), our librarian sends a message to our inner security system, which activates our threat response and we rapidly prepare for action.

This security system is sometimes referred to as being monkey-like, owing to the primitive nature of the response – emotional rather than logical. Once activated, it begins to influence how we think, feel and behave, causing us to make choices and take actions to deal with the threat, which may be real or imagined, physical or psychological. We then experience the adapted thoughts, feelings and behaviours as symptoms or problems, which may create undesirable, stressful outcomes in our lives (4b), until the perceived or imagined threat has passed.

Following this Library Model in order to make changes then, there are three main areas we can focus on:

- Managing the symptoms arising from our inner security response
- Changing the beliefs and ideas triggering it in the first place
- Reframing the memories and stored information that formed the beliefs via natural hypnosis

All therapy or self-help will fall into one or more of these categories and any time we can be successful in addressing our issues in one or more of these ways, we can experience positive change.

Managing the symptoms can be an ongoing task, however, like facing never-ending zombies in a zombie movie or continually mopping the floor from an overflowing basin. Dealing with the underlying beliefs and/or memories will create a deeper, more lasting result as we effectively de-hypnotize ourselves from what we have been thinking and feeling, like defeating the zombie master or pulling out the plug and switching off the tap.

There is a challenge to overcome, though, because in order to sort out the underlying causes, we often have to face up to things we would rather not, and that in itself triggers our security response, often making us avoid or resist that final step. We can revert to trying to instil positive ideas instead, but very often they too trigger the security response.

We can even try to avoid the source of our issues entirely. But, alas, we unwittingly seem to seek them out anyway, or life finds a way of throwing them at us, until we face up to them. Whatever happens, if we wish to evolve and become a better, happier version of ourselves, we do eventually have to face up to any ideas holding us back and resolve any internal conflicts.

The good news is, however, we needn't be scared. Although it can seem difficult at first, on the other side of fear is freedom – and that is where we are heading.

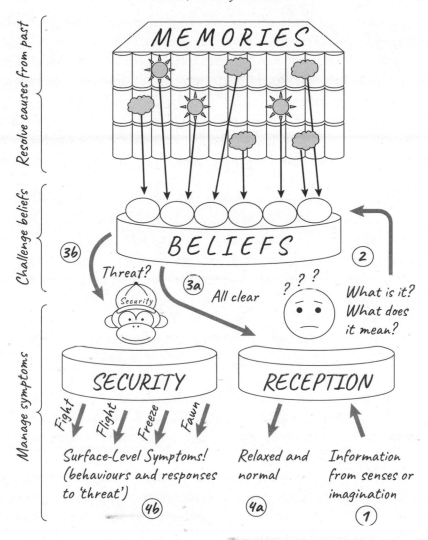

The Missing Ingredient That Will Finally Work For You

To me, any period of growth or change will require a combination of work with ourselves and an interaction with others. While we can do an awful lot ourselves, sometimes we just need another person to interact with in order to bring out the ideas and beliefs that are invisible to us – largely because of the way *we protect ourselves from going there*.

I was chatting to a lady recently about weight loss and she suddenly acknowledged that there was a disconnect in her mind between what went into her mouth and what went into her body.

'In my mind, the food goes no further than here,' she said, placing her hand at throat level. 'It's as if I just cannot see or acknowledge that the food goes any further.'

When I pushed her on this and persisted with the questioning, both fear and shame came up. It was this fear and shame that she had been protecting herself from feeling – both in her daily behaviours and in her self-therapy.

Sometimes we just need someone to help us notice these things or to help us see beyond the limitations of our own beliefs and the fight or flight adaptive behaviours that come from those.

To me, the missing ingredient that will finally make self-help work for you is that . . . **sometimes we actually need someone else's help! And that is OK!**

I have often noticed that my expressing this casually on training courses has generated a great sigh of relief from many people as they released their guilt for not being 'fixed' after reading a certain book.

Sometimes we just need someone to interact with who can reflect ourselves back to us or help us access those deeper levels. This may be a paid professional, a trusted friend or anyone we can have a meaningful conversation with. Sometimes even a difficult 'enemy' can be the trigger we need, if we are willing to face up to what we are feeling and have those difficult conversations with them. But whichever way it happens, we very often need that human interaction to trigger the threat response, so that the invisible becomes visible, the underlying fear or upset is brought to the surface, and we can then do something about it.

Does solving personal problems and transforming our lives always have to involve such deep probing and questioning in order to make progress?

Not at all.

Are there other ways, including things we can do ourselves, that actually work?

Absolutely. But it all depends on what we are seeking to achieve and at what level we need to bring about change in order to do that.

As we progress through the book we will explore different areas that you can work on yourself and those where you may need assistance, and give further examples of how you can consciously create the conditions for positive change in yourself. But rather than seeing these issues as annoying problems to be resolved so you can get on with life, I would like to suggest a new vision for personal transformation, a way of thinking that seems to fit in more with a wider picture of our species as a whole.

A New Vision for Personal Transformation

If we want to get from overweight to slim and stay there, something has to change. If we want to get from self-sabotage and failure to allowing success, something has to change. If we want to get from difficult relationships to loving relationships, something has to change. If we want to get from stress and anxiety to calm and confident, something has to change. If we want to get from low self-worth and low self-esteem to feeling valued and worthy, and stay there, something has to change. These are the kinds of issues I have been helping people with for nearly thirty years now. If we want to get from any state of being to another *and stay there*, something has to change – usually a fundamental shift in our belief system.

Following a fundamental shift in our belief system we will have different thoughts that create different feelings that allow us to make different choices and create different behaviours – all of which will bring about more desirable outcomes and results.

Nothing can make us into something we are not, but by overcoming life challenges in this way, we most certainly evolve as a person and become something more.

So instead of asking, 'How can I fix this problem or make this issue go away?', I believe we should be asking these questions:

- Who do I need to become in order to evolve from this so that this is no longer a pattern in my life?
- What will that more evolved version of myself look and feel like?
- What beliefs does this more evolved version of me carry, so that I can begin to adopt and incorporate them now?

- What old identity do I need to let go of in order to allow a more evolved identity to take its place?
- What fears must I face up to?
- What positive attributes in myself must I finally recognize and allow to be a gift to the world?
- What can I do myself?
- Where might I need some help?
- What needs to happen for me to truly live and love my life – and more importantly, myself?

The remainder of this book is designed to help you achieve the answers to these questions. Whether it takes years, months, weeks, days, hours, minutes or seconds, you can escape the fears and perceived limitations of your life. You can finally unlock the Real You and become the person you were born to be.

PART TWO

The E.S.C.A.P.E. Method

What is the E.S.C.A.P.E. Method?

The E.S.C.A.P.E. Method is a set of thought exercises, questions and responses that, if followed with honesty and persistence, will help you get from where you are to where you want to be.

Each of the letters will reveal a key to unlocking more of the Real You, and take you, step by step, closer to feeling lighter, freer and more unburdened from life. The key areas are:

Enoughness
Safeness
Control
Acceptance
Pleasure, and finally
En-lightenment

It is not always easy doing this by yourself though, for reasons explained earlier. You will probably resist at times. You will probably feel as if you have failed at times. You will probably find yourself back at the bottom of that escalator at times, with the top still looking a very long way up. All that is normal and to be expected. That is life. That is the nature of personal transformation.

However, I absolutely 100 per cent guarantee and promise that if you *are* persistent and willing to do what is required, the more desirable circumstances and transformations in personal, emotional and behavioural areas of your life that you wish for are there for the asking . . . though the means of achieving them and the form they take when they arrive may not always be how you have imagined them until now.

As you embark on this journey, you will need to let go of any expectations as to how you think it should be and instead let it unfold for you. Remember, it is not about the journey or the destination, it is about *who you become* on the way that will bring you greater happiness, and this is a lifelong process with many chapters, full of twists and turns, often arising when we least expect them.

Remember, also, that every challenge or problem is an opportunity in disguise – an opportunity to recognize a fear, identify a limiting belief, to evolve beyond it and become something more.

Right now, there are areas of life you wish to change – even if you are unsure exactly what they are. Some of those things may be 'out there' in the world, relating to physical situations or circumstances; others will be more 'inner desires', relating to how you think or feel. Either way, there will also be reasons why you want to change them – things you no longer want to feel, things you would rather feel instead – and the changes you desire are a means for achieving that. Some of these may be well thought out; others may be acts of desperation triggered by the threat response discussed earlier.

Single-minded determination and focus can go a long way to helping us achieve things, but also bear in mind this saying:

> *Never be so sure of what you want that you are*
> *unwilling to be open to something even better.*

As you begin this journey, it can seem as if you begin it alone, reading the words on these pages, applying the exercises as best you can. But, instead, imagine that a voice is with you: helping you, guiding you, encouraging you, supporting you, reassuring you. Imagine that voice is the you that has already completed this journey and is now sending back encouragement and clues as to how to achieve the same level of success, happiness and contentment, this future you have.

Besides that inner voice, you may need outside help as well, at times. **That is OK!** That help may be in the form of a trusted friend, an E.S.C.A.P.E. Buddy, a paid professional or simply 'life' sending conditions your way that are forcing you to face up to something. As you will see, there are times when we just need someone or something else to bounce ideas off or stop us in our tracks to make sure that we pay attention. We can especially enlist the help of our own subconscious mind at times as well, which I will also show you how to do.

The future you is already within you and actually no different to who you are right now. This process is less about something you need to become and more about something you already are but just need to *set free*: the Real You, the one who has been hiding under layers of fears and limitations until now.

This is why I call it the E.S.C.A.P.E. Method – application of the exercises and principles that follow will help to dehypnotize you from the fears and limitations that have effectively imprisoned you in certain areas, and escape, so that you can finally unlock the Real You and be free.

What You Will Need

The main thing you will need is a simple willingness to face up to things – everything else kind of takes care of itself after that. But there are some practical aids you can employ as well.

Journal

I would suggest you get yourself a nice journal, something that feels special when you pick it up, something precious. It doesn't need to be expensive, but it does need to stand out or mean something to you.

Pen

I would also suggest you get a nice pen to use. Again, it doesn't need to be expensive, just something that means a little bit extra to you each time you pick it up, something that will act as a symbol of connection to what you wish to achieve.

Time

You will need to set aside time to do some of these exercises. For some, just a few minutes a day will suffice. As we progress, you may wish to block out longer periods of fifteen to twenty minutes, or even an hour or so for some of the more detailed ones.

There is no set time of day to do these – just whatever works best for you, when you can find a quiet and peaceful moment to reflect on the ideas we are presenting. Some will prefer mornings, some will prefer evenings, and others would rather wait until the weekend. All of these are OK, there are no rules and there is no time limit or time pressure.

Space

You will actually be using many of the exercises as you go through your day in your everyday environment, but for the more structured exercises, you will find it more beneficial if you can find a quiet and peaceful place where the conditions are best for self-reflection.

You do not need to go to great lengths for this, just somewhere where you will not be disturbed and can relax a while. Ideally somewhere quiet, free of distractions, so that you can be aware of your thoughts as they arise.

Support

Depending upon the areas of life you are seeking to make changes in, you may need the support of those around you, including family and friends. Sometimes this will be for encouragement; sometimes it may be that you simply need to warn them that you are going through something and to cut you a little slack for a while.

This does not mean we are free to use someone close to us as an emotional punchbag, but instead as someone you can be brave enough to express your fears to – which is often all we need do once we identify them, as you will see.

Again, your E.S.C.A.P.E. Buddy, which I explain in a moment, may come in handy here as well.

Rest and Recovery

You cannot force this and will need to incorporate periods of rest and recovery. If you find yourself struggling or straining with the exercises, walk away, take a break, get some sleep. Our brains literally get overloaded and need periods of rest to file away what is useful and dispose of what is not.

This is not about running up that down escalator – it is about stopping it from being a down escalator and turning it into an up escalator. Sleep, rest and periods of recovery are vital for this.

Patience

Many of us will put off what we need to do to make changes, but when we finally make the decision to go for it, we want it done *now*!

Sometimes that is OK and will drive us forward; other times we may need to be patient and allow things to fall into place. From experience, personal growth will involve periods of activity followed by periods of integration and assimilation, during which we may need to exercise a great deal of patience.

As long as we can discern between patience and avoidance, it is perfectly OK to allow things to fall into place for a while. But if we sense we are avoiding, that is the time to instead face the fears and take action.

Using an E.S.C.A.P.E. Buddy

All of these exercises are designed for you to do yourself, but there are times when you may find it helpful to enlist the services of a trusted friend or family member to bounce ideas off or to ask you certain questions.

It is vital that you only choose someone you trust, who is kind and supportive to you – but at the same time, you do not want to change the balance of your friendship or relationship by turning them into your therapist! Ideally, you should buddy up with someone who is interested in going through the process as well, and as you swap roles, you will maintain the balance.

If you do use an E.S.C.A.P.E. Buddy then it is important to keep your roles separate. Most people find this difficult because as soon as someone starts to speak, we immediately relate it to ourselves and want to talk about ourselves or give advice. In conversation, that's fine. In this process, that's a no-no!

If you are playing the role of the Buddy to someone else, the session should be focused on that someone else, not a two-way discussion. And then, when it is your turn to receive the help, the session should be focused on you.

Also, as a Buddy, *it is not your job to give advice or solve the problem*. You are there to help your fellow *escapee* gather information, so your main roles are to look out for *unfinished sentences* and ask what I call *Fluid Questions*, as explained below, to keep the information flowing.

Unfinished Sentences

One day I suddenly noticed how clients would often stop mid-sentence and go off at a tangent. And the inquisitive part of me was wondering what they were about to say but didn't – or what they avoided! What had they 'resisted' telling me?

The typical convention in counselling and therapy is to let the client speak and to not interrupt, but once I had picked up on this, I decided to ignore the convention, interrupt their avoidance tactic and take them back to finish the sentence – with profound results. Practically every time I did that, there would be a useful nugget of information in there – and often clients would suddenly break down and have emotional outpourings on the spot, many times revealing the true, hidden cause of their issue that they had never told anybody.

It might go something like this:

CLIENT: When I was a child I was very – well, Mum and Dad used to work a lot and didn't often get home until late.

ME: What were you about to say? 'When I was a child I was very . . .'?

CLIENT: Nothing, it's just that –

ME: Go on, finish that sentence. 'When I was a child I was very . . .'?

CLIENT: Lonely. I was very lonely. [Gets upset.]

The avoided word would then open up a whole new line of enquiry, and very often a deep, instant and profound transformation would occur, often to the surprise of the subject.

So much of what we need to face up to is actually really close to the surface, when you know how to look. If you work with people in any kind of personal capacity, have them finish their unfinished sentences and see what comes out. And for yourself, pay attention to any time you stop a sentence mid-flow and change tack. Pay attention to what you were *about* to say but didn't – there will be something in that!

Unfinished sentences – and unfinished words because we may even break off mid-word – will often reveal unfinished business. And the reason we do not want to finish the sentence or word is because, if we do, it will take us closer to the feeling of the unfinished business we do not want to feel. The threat response kicks in, we stop what we are about to say and say something else instead, thereby temporarily avoiding or escaping the issue, leaving our invisible, limiting belief intact to live another day and subconsciously influence us when the next opportunity arises. From my experience, many cases of stuttering and stammering are extreme versions of this, where the process has become subconscious and automatic.

Fluid Questions

At my Practitioner Academy, where I train people in the methods I use so that they can then help others, there's an exercise I give my students that they usually find very difficult. I give them a sheet of paper containing a list of questions and ask them to initiate a conversation with a fellow student acting as the client, but they – the one playing the therapist – are only allowed to respond to what the other says by asking one of the questions on that sheet.

It's amazing to see the frustration, the difficulty, of not being able to give an opinion, offer advice or relate an experience of their own. I ask them to keep this going for around ten minutes, while the 'client' talks on a subject of their choice, usually something light-hearted initially.

The questions seem innocent but are designed to encourage the subject to probe deeper into their mind, searching for answers, beyond the protection of the critical faculty, without realizing they are doing so. The client still has the opportunity to filter what they say, of course – but when we add in picking up on unfinished sentences or unfinished words, the client soon finds themselves backed into a corner, revealing more and more information in what feels a very conversational manner, yet reaches very deep. I put a great deal of emphasis on mastering this skill.

This process works well enough conversationally, but when we do it in a relaxed and inwardly focused state like natural hypnosis, the effect is often dramatically multiplied. The reduced distraction from external stimuli allows the inner thoughts and ideas to more readily come to the surface and the increased focus means we are less able to pretend they are not there (i.e. 'resist' them), if we're not keen on going there at first.

This is how and why we can often get to the core of issues more directly than when using the more traditional methods.

As we have discussed already, we are all actually very good at protecting ourselves from going to where we need to, but when we have a conversation in the right way – i.e. being asked probing questions – it gets a little trickier to do that. Ideally, we would have these conversations with a trained professional, but sometimes a structured chat with a good friend or someone we trust can be equally helpful, as can a conversation with ourselves.

Remember though, when working with a Buddy, if you are the one asking the questions, you are asking questions – not offering a solution, opinion, advice or telling your own story!

See if you can get into the habit of using these questions:

- In what way?
- What's that like?
- Is there anything else?

Let's call the person wanting to resolve something the 'Escapee' and the person helping them out is the Buddy. So the conversation could go something like this:

ESCAPEE: I need some confidence for swimming.
BUDDY: In what way?
ESCAPEE: I get nervous.
BUDDY: What kind of nervous?

ESCAPEE: Like I am going to suddenly get tired and not be able to continue.

BUDDY: In what way?

ESCAPEE: Like I'll just get short of breath and not be able to make it.

BUDDY: And what's *that* like?

ESCAPEE: It's dange– I don't know.

BUDDY: Finish that word, 'It's dange . . .'

ESCAPEE: It's dangerous – I'll feel out of control and helpless, so I get scared even going in.

BUDDY: Is there anything else?

ESCAPEE: Yes, this happened when I was a child, and I have never felt the same since. It was deeper than I thought and I shouldn't have been swimming there. I got really scared and out of breath, and didn't think I was going to make it to the other side.

This is an abbreviated version of the actual discussion, and the mention of the bad experience may even trigger some emotion – again one of the reasons why this questioning gets to the root so quickly – but at this point we now have some information to work with.

The Buddy system should never be used when the person needs more professional help, such as dealing with major traumas or clinical depression, for example, but for everyday fears, worries and anxieties, you will be surprised at how easy it can sometimes be to get a shift in perspective and an easing of symptoms.

And if someone gets upset or tearful, it's OK, just be reassuring. It will eventually pass and they may then decide to request a session with someone trained in this to help resolve whatever the deeper upset is. There are more details on this in the 'Next Step' section at the back of the book (p. 319).

How Long Will It Take?

To bring about consistent change in any particular area, it will take as long as it takes for your beliefs and behaviours to consistently shift in that particular area. In some areas, a simple word or phrase may instantly give you the shift in perspective needed to free you from an old limitation and create immediate results; in other areas, there may be a lifetime of conditioning to undo, full of emotionally charged memories and life experiences that need to be healed.

The simple answer is, it will take as long as it takes, but the more time you can dedicate to this, the more likely you are to speed up the process. However, as a guide, anybody who employs the exercises with full openness and persistence should experience initial benefits within thirty days or less.

That is not a promise of 'Your Life Completely Sorted In Thirty Days' – but there should be some perceivable shift so that you can feel you are making progress, which you can then develop further by delving deeper. Longer term benefits will then follow.

What Areas Can We Use This On?

These are some of the common areas I have helped people with:

- Anxiety and Confidence
- Alcohol, Drugs and Addictions
- Diets and Weight Loss
- Eating Disorders
- Health and Fitness
- Pain Relief
- Sports and Performance
- Ageing
- Sex and Intimacy
- Business, Work, Career and Wealth
- Love and Relationships
- Public Speaking and Speech Issues
- Pregnancy and Fertility
- Habits

And so many more.

In fact, anything where our thoughts, feelings, emotions and behaviours are involved!

Will you feel differently after following these suggestions? I don't know you well enough yet to know how well you will put them into practice. However, I do know that they can and will be extremely transformative when applied in the right way. I have witnessed it in myself and many thousands of times in the people I have worked with. It can work for you too.

Success and Failure

I know it is tempting to try to protect ourselves from this particular F word, but somebody once told me, 'It doesn't matter how much perfume you use, you cannot make a piece of dog poop smell nice!'

If ever we do not achieve success – i.e. a desired outcome – in something, in that moment it is perfectly OK to acknowledge that, technically, we have 'failed' – this time, in this way.

Failure is a part of everyday life and should be treated and accepted as such. Sometimes it's not much of a big deal, sometimes it is a very big deal. Sometimes we can brush it off. Sometimes it hurts like hell.

The only problem with failure is if we let it define us and start thinking, 'I *am* a failure,' because that will then leave us back at the bottom of the moving staircase, looking up, scared to try again.

If we fail it means we have not achieved our desired outcome that time, in that way. That's all. Every super-successful person will have a string of failures under their belt, things that didn't work out the way they planned. Have you ever seen those nature programmes where the lions' prey gets away, leaving the pride still hungry and panting with exhaustion? Or a top sports person missing a goal or flunking a shot? We all fail at times.

I once ran an online webinar, paid for advertising, sent out the emails, took a couple of days writing the content, set aside a whole Sunday to prepare . . . and not a single person showed up. Not one. I did the webinar anyway, to myself, starting on time, presenting for the hour, chatting away, just in case someone turned up late. But no one did.

Was it a failure? Absolutely! Completely! Utterly! No amount of perfume can disguise that. Did I achieve what I set out to achieve? Nowhere even close.

Did it make *me* a failure? No. I felt pretty rubbish for a while and *felt* like a failure, but did I learn anything from it? You bet!

The only thing wrong with failing is if we keep doing the same thing again and again and never learn. (Though I have done that quite a lot too!) As long as we learn something from it (eventually) – and by that I typically mean what caused it and what *not* to do next time – then failure can be a great teacher.

I'm not saying we should go around failing on purpose in order to grow, that would be rather pointless; or even that we should too easily accept failure and give up. But if we avoid things because we are scared of failure, we may also be scared of doing the things that will ultimately teach us how to be successful.

If you have failed at helping yourself with this sort of thing in the past, it's OK. It probably just means you either didn't have the right information or life had somehow set you up to not be able to use it in the right way yet. Give yourself a break.

You will experience what at first seems like failure, but if you can learn from it, eventually you will experience success.

Harness the qualities of *persistence* and *resilience*. These are the best friends of success. With these in our arsenal we are able to go again, make a fresh start, pick ourselves up and get on with it, however many times it takes to get where we want to be.

Questions Must Be Answered

One last thing before we get started: all questions must be answered. Or in other words, 'I don't know' is not allowed! Sometimes 'I don't know' actually means 'I don't want to know' or 'I know but I don't want to say'. Other times, it may just take a while for an answer to come to the surface. If you find yourself thinking, 'I don't know,' that's OK at first, but then dig deep, ask for help if you need it or take a break to think about it, but you must find an answer and the answer must ultimately feel true to you. This is the only way to get past resistance and access the Real You.

OK, time to get on with it.

Exercise 1: Awareness of Meaning

Duration: 5–10 minutes
Journal Required: Yes
Buddy Required: No

Background

The first thing we need to understand if we are to be successful in creating change is that we give meaning to everything we encounter. The meaning we give it will determine how we feel, respond or react, which will determine the outcomes we experience. If we give it a good meaning, we typically feel good; if we give it a bad meaning, we typically feel bad. The meaning we give things comes from our beliefs and our beliefs are formed from life experiences – our past.

So we could say we are rarely seeing things as they are; instead, we are seeing things as symbols of our past, which our mind will attempt to replay.

This very first mindfulness exercise is to help you become aware of that, so that you can begin the process of dehypnotizing yourself from conditioned meanings and responses.*

Please do not be tempted to rush this – take your time and give

* I first learned about attaching meanings from *A Course in Miracles* (scribed by Helen Schucman) and these exercises are my own adaptations from that.

it your full attention. In a way, this simple exercise holds the key to freedom from many of our issues . . .

Instructions

Part 1

1. Find a quiet place where you will not be disturbed for a few minutes.
2. Take at least five or six long, slow, deep breaths to allow yourself to slow down, relax and focus. Making your out-breath longer than your in-breath will help to simulate a feeling of relief and encourage your parasympathetic nervous system to keep the threat response deactivated for a while.
3. Set a timer for two minutes on your phone.
4. For the entire duration of those two minutes, look around you and allow your eyes to fall on the different objects you see.
5. For each one, remind yourself of the label you give it, and remind yourself that there is a meaning you attach to it (i.e. what it is, what we do with it, how we use it, what it means to us).

For example, as I look around the room where I am writing this:

- I see an extension lead . . . and I attach a meaning to it.
- I see an electric guitar . . . and I attach a meaning to it.
- I see a door handle on a cupboard . . . and I attach a meaning to it.
- I see a cupboard . . . and I attach a meaning to it.
- I see a garden spade through the window . . . and I attach a meaning to it.
- I see a table in the corner . . . and I attach a meaning to it.
- I see wood panelling on the walls . . . and I attach a meaning to it.
- I see my hand . . . and I attach a meaning to it.
- I see a light switch . . . and I attach a meaning to it.

Repeat this for everything and anything your gaze falls upon. It is vital that you do not pick and choose anything over anything else – all must be treated equally. You do *not* need to write this down.

If you do this slowly and with enough focus, you will begin to notice that each item you focus on will trigger a response. Assuming the objects are familiar to you, you will know what they are and what they are for . . . but on top of this, your mind may even trigger flashes of memory relating to when you last used the items or imaginings of when you may do so in the future.

As you do this exercise, I want you to become consciously aware of the process that usually happens subconsciously. You are identifying objects and attaching a meaning as your subconscious pulls up memories or imaginings for you.

Do not proceed further until you have done this.

Part 2

Once you have completed Part 1, either take a break for a few moments or carry on to this stage later in the day if you wish.

When you are ready, repeat the exercise, but this time with your eyes closed, using your *imagination* and relating it to different *people* in your life.

1. Find a quiet place where you will not be disturbed for a few minutes.
2. Set a timer for two minutes.
3. Take a few long, slow, deep breaths to allow yourself to relax and allow your out-breaths to be longer than your in-breaths, as before, so that they feel more like sighs of relief and your body can relax.
4. Start the timer and allow your eyes to close.
5. For the entire duration of those two minutes, allow your mind to think of different people in your life.
6. For each one, remind yourself of the label you give that person and also become aware of any meaning you attach to them.

Again, do not pick and choose – if someone comes to mind, apply the exercise to them. For example:

- I am thinking of my neighbour . . . and I attach a meaning to this person.
- I am thinking of my son/daughter . . . and I attach a meaning to this person.
- I am thinking of my partner . . . and I attach a meaning to this person.
- I am thinking of the stranger who pulled out in front of me earlier . . . and I attach a meaning to this person.
- I am thinking of the person who served me in the shop yesterday . . . and I attach a meaning to this person.

If you do this persistently, for the entire two minutes, and you allow each person who comes to mind to be treated equally, you will most likely also begin to experience some feelings and emotions – i.e. emotive meanings.

Part 3

In your journal make a note of as many of those people who came to mind as you can and beside each one write either:

- 'P' for a positive feeling/meaning
- 'F' for a negative feeling/meaning
- 'M' if there was a mixture of positive and negative
- 'N' if there was a completely neutral feeling/meaning

(You may be wondering why 'F' for negative – I will explain later.)

By doing this, you are again making a subconscious process become conscious, and becoming aware of any emotive meanings you have been applying to people. These emotive meanings will actually be indicators of your beliefs.

More on that to follow, but you can now begin to play with this exercise any time you think of it as you go through your day. Just observe yourself noticing things and say, 'I am attaching a meaning to this,' and in your encounters with people, again, observe any feelings or reactions you experience, saying, 'I am attaching a meaning to this person.'

Advanced Version

If you wish to progress further, do this exercise every day for a week.

If you wish to progress further still, choose a day and repeat this exercise every four hours. Then do it again the next day. And the next.

Then choose a day and repeat it every hour. Then every half hour. You do not need to write everything down every time, if you choose to do these more extreme versions, but pausing every hour for two minutes to settle back and become aware of everything in your surroundings, everything running through your mind and the meanings you are currently giving to everything will dramatically accelerate your awareness. And you may actually be able to step back from it a little, which will also help reduce any build-up of stress or tension that may be there.

Now, let's get a bit more specific . . .

Exercise 2: 3-2-1 Analysis Practice

Duration: 10–15 minutes
Journal Required: Yes
Buddy Required: Optional

Background

As human beings, we often focus too much on the negatives in life, without appreciating the positives; or, conversely, focus too much on the positives, while avoiding facing up to the things that we need to face up to. I'd like to help instil a new habit in you that will allow you to become more positively focused, while at the same time allowing you to deal with any negatives or areas of concern.

It is a model for self-reflection, and takes the form of:

- Three things about [A] that [X]
- Two things about [A] that [Y]
- One thing about [A] that [Z]

In a teaching scenario, it could be:

- Three things about a certain topic I found interesting
- Two things about the topic I would like to research further
- One thing about the topic I need clarification on

After hearing this applied to sports performance, I also began using it to great effect with sports people I was working with, discussing individual and team performances after a game. For example:

- Three things I did well [today/this week/this month]
- Two things I would like to improve upon
- One thing I would like to change immediately

For our exercise here, we are going to use it to help you focus on:

- Three areas that are good in life
- Two areas that you would *like* or *want* to change
- One area that *needs* to change

Instructions

Part 1

Think about your life as a whole and, on a new page in your journal, write the heading '3-2-1 Analysis Practice'. Underneath that, write down:

- Three things that you feel are good or positive about your life (i.e. three things that you give a positive meaning to)
- Two things that you would like to change or improve
- One thing that you feel NEEDS to change right now, even if you are reluctant to face up to it

Go with whatever comes to mind for now and whichever area of life you think of first, but **stick to the 3-2-1** – we do not want a great long list! This is just to practise doing the exercise.

If you can write down three positive things, great. If you struggle, you must persist until you can. If you need help, ask someone you trust to give you some ideas. Whatever you do, do not skip this. Stay with it until you can write down three positive things about your life. You must do this, even if it is as basic as 'I have a bed to sleep in, I have a roof over my head, I have some food to eat.'

Part 2

Focus on these three positive statements and read them aloud if you can.

They must be *true* or *feel true* when you say them. Make sure you are not quoting some generic positive-thinking-type statement you have read somewhere – make it real, authentic, using everyday words from your everyday vocabulary.

These positives will form the foundation of what happens next. Every time you can read them or say them to yourself, knowing they are true or feel true, you will be reinforcing them – via natural hypnosis – allowing them to reinforce your conscious beliefs and go deep into your subconscious for reference.

This is why they must be *true*. We do not want that critical faculty acting as gatekeeper – we want these ideas allowed in. If they are true, they will be, because there should be little or no resistance.

Test this out – I want you to know and recognize what it feels like when you are affirming positive ideas to yourself. I want you to notice how your body feels when you are saying positive things *that are true* to yourself. You are not trying to prove anything to anybody or convince anybody of anything. You are just stating it, like it is.

I also want you to look out for any conflict within you – one part of you knowing these ideas are true and yet something somewhere feeling resistant or reactive to them – as if consciously you know and believe one thing but subconsciously there is something reacting against the idea. If you sense a conflict, for now, choose a different statement instead, one where there is no conflict or resistance.

In your journal, write down a few words that describe:

1. What it feels like when you say something positive about yourself or your life that you know to be true.
2. What it feels like when there is resistance or conflict, if you felt that (which may be inner self-talk or sensations in your body, for example).

Part 3

Now, look at the two things you would like to change, and the one thing that you feel 'needs' to change.

The two things you would like to change will probably give you superficial benefits; the one thing that needs to change will probably bring you a deeper transformation. They may or may not be connected, but they often are at some level, and dealing with the one thing that needs to change will often also help to bring about changes in the other areas as well.

Think about this in your example above, and in your journal make a note of what you think the impact would be on the 'two things', if you could only sort out the 'one thing'.

Good. Take a break, then when you are ready, move on to the next exercise.

Exercise 3: Your Wishlist

Duration: 30–60 minutes
Journal Required: Yes
Buddy Required: Optional

Background

In the world of sales and marketing, people often talk about products and services being divided into three main niches or categories:

- Health and Well-being
- Career and Money
- Relationships and Intimacy

This makes sense because these cover pretty much every area of our lives. There is often a fourth area around spirituality, but I'll come to that later. For now, I want you to think about each of these three main areas and do a 3-2-1 analysis of each one.

Why all of them? Because if you didn't have to do all of them, you would possibly avoid the ones you are resistant to. If any part of you is scared to go there, the threat response will subtly activate, you will feel uncomfortable and then find a logical, rational reason as to why you do not need to do so right now.

Don't be fooled! Remember, resistance is futile and will only delay the process. It doesn't mean you have to suddenly leap into life-changing decisions; it does mean you can resolve the fear around them, so that when or if you have to make a decision, you can do so from a better place. So let's do all three areas to make sure you are getting the absolute maximum benefit.

Instructions

Part 1 – Health and Well-being

1. Take a page in your journal and write the heading 'Health and Well-being' at the top of the page. You may wish to word it slightly differently if it feels better to do so.
2. Think about things that relate to the general health and well-being of your body: health conditions, fitness, weight, diet, exercise, sleep – all come under this category.
3. Do a 3-2-1 analysis of your current situation, writing down:

   - Three positive statements about your current health and well-being situation
   - Two areas where there is room for improvement or you would like to make changes
   - One area where you really need to make a change

4. Read each of your answers back to yourself. The three positives should feel true and give you a positive foundation on which to start. The two things you'd like to change should give you positive feelings about the idea of changing them. And the one thing that *needs* to change should feel awesome if that could only be sorted out, even if there is fear or hesitation involved right now, or you do not know how yet.
5. For each of the 'two things' and the 'one thing', give yourself a score out of 10 for how motivated you feel about making these changes right now, where 10 = *very* and 0 = *not at all*.

Be sure to avoid any intellectualization or worry about how to make the changes – just identify the areas by doing the 3-2-1 analysis, give yourself a current motivation score and then move on to Part 2.

Part 2 – Career and Money

1. Take a page in your journal and write the heading 'Career and Money' at the top of the page. Again, you may wish to word it slightly differently if it feels better to do so.
2. Think about things that relate to the areas of your life around work, career and money: job satisfaction, education, finances, workload, promotions, savings, debts, possessions, etc., can all come under this category.
3. Follow steps 3, 4 and 5 as above.

Again, be sure to avoid any overthinking or worry about how to make the changes – just identify the areas first of all, give yourself a score, take a break if you need it, and then move on to Part 3.

Part 3 – Relationships and Intimacy

1. Take a page in your journal and write the heading 'Relationships and Intimacy' at the top of the page, or reword if you prefer to make it more specific to a chosen area.
2. Think about things that relate to the areas of your life around Relationships and Intimacy: significant other, family, children, friends, colleagues, sex, dating, closeness, fun and socializing can all come under this category.
3. Follow steps 3, 4 and 5 as above.

Again, be sure to avoid any overintellectualization or worry about how to make the changes – just identify the areas first of all, give yourself a score and then move on to Part 4.

Part 4

Now read aloud what you have written for Parts 1–3 of this exercise, in a format something like this:

In the area of Health and Well-being, three good things I can build on now are the facts that [Positive 1, Positive 2 and Positive 3]. I would really like to change [your two areas you would like to change], and it would be awesome [you can use a different word if you wish!] if I could change [your one thing that needs to change].

In the area of Career and Money, three good things I can build on now are the facts that [Positive 1, Positive 2 and Positive 3]. I would really like to change [your two areas you would like to change], and it would be awesome if I could change [your one thing that needs to change].

In the area of Relationships and Intimacy, three good things I can build on now are the facts that [Positive 1, Positive 2 and Positive 3]. I would really like to change [your two areas you would like to change], and it would be awesome if I could change [your one thing that needs to change].

Pay attention to how you *feel* as you read through all of this. That future you, who has already achieved this, should be calling to you. The Real You – the one inside who has been hiding until now – should be beginning to stir. And your critical faculty will be watching closely, to check it is safe . . .

Are You Interested or Are You Committed?

I don't know who created this question initially but it will usually help separate those of us who are likely to succeed in getting to where we want to get to and those who are not. Those who are interested may have dreams and goals but never do anything, whereas those who are committed will take the actions required to get there.

Interested will talk about changing things; committed will actually do so. Interested walks down the sidewalk, falls in the hole, says, 'Ouch, no way I am doing that again,' and heads back to safety; committed keeps going, sometimes falling into hole after hole, but learning on the way, until they eventually manage to avoid the holes and achieve success – whatever that may be.

In these areas of life you want to change, it will often take much more than a passing interest to bring about successful transformation – it will usually take quite a degree of commitment.

That doesn't mean we have to slog away day and night with no sleep until we get there. Of course, there are times when that sort of commitment is required to complete a task, and in such cases it is only the commitment to the result that will encourage us to see it through, long after we may be tempted to quit. But seeking to bring about any kind of change in our life will require a degree of persistence – and it is *commitment* to the result, the outcome, that will enable that persistence.

So as we think about these areas of life we are seeking to transform, we must ask ourselves, 'Am I interested or am I committed?'

There's no right or wrong, by the way. It's up to you. And it's OK if you start with 'interested' and see where it takes you. I have had many people express their interest in getting help from me or taking one of my courses for several years before they finally act. Their interest keeps bringing them back, but often it takes a certain set of circumstances or certain timing for them to cross that threshold from interested to committed.

And that's fine. It has to be when the time is right, and that essentially boils down to another factor we haven't yet discussed.

I remember giving a short talk to the Lewes FC Women's Football Team. At the time of writing they are the first and only football/soccer club in the world to pay their women the same as their men. I thought that was a worthy cause to donate some time to and began chatting with various players to see if I could help them improve performance, both on and off the pitch.

At that first talk, I explained, 'As a team, what you actually *do* is up here,' holding my hands at about head height. 'Underneath that are your beliefs and values, which help determine *how* you do that,' I went on, holding my hands at about chest height. 'But deep down here –' I held my hands at belly-button height – 'there is one more level that acts as the foundation for all of this and everything else. Can anybody tell me what that is?' I asked hopefully.

I looked around in silence at twenty pairs of eyes, some looking at me, some avoiding my gaze, until eventually someone spoke up. 'Why?' said New Zealand international Katie 'Roodie' Rood.

'Yes!' I said thankfully, relieved that someone had responded. 'Why!'

There are many, many books on this topic, but one of the best ways to really get a feel for it is to watch the TED Talk by Simon Sinek, which is where I got this idea of three levels from: *What – How – Why.*

'What you do is up here,' I repeated, 'how you do it is here, and why is deep down here, almost in your guts – and that is what I usually need to dig into if we are going to elevate your performance and bring out the best in you.'

Whenever *anybody* asks me to help them make a change in some way, underneath the whole pile of information they give, what I really want to know is *Why?* Why bother? Why not just stay the way you are? Why do you want to get rid of this problem? Why do you want something else instead? What is that something else you want? What is it you want to achieve? Why? Why? Why?! Not having a big enough 'Why' is often one of the reasons we remain stuck. In such cases we often know that we should change and may even actually want to change, but if we do not have a big enough reason to change now, today, we may end up putting it off and procrastinating (freeze response) until we do have a big enough reason.

I remember a friend of mine who smoked 20–40 cigarettes a day walking up to me on the dance floor at a mutual friend's wedding and shouting in my ear that I needed to help him stop smoking.

I thought for a moment. I knew this person was an avid record collector, passionate about music. 'Just imagine how many records you could buy if you didn't smoke,' I said, and he stepped back and smiled.

Catching up with him nearly twenty years later, he reminded me of the story and told me he had never smoked a single cigarette since that evening.

It is the 'Why' that will create interest in change. It is having a big enough 'Why' that will help us stay committed with enough persistence to see that change through to completion.

However, the 'Why' that gets us interested and the 'Why' that gets us committed may not always be the same. As with my friend, health got him interested in quitting smoking, but being able to buy more records got him committed to doing so!

Towards and Away From Motivation

We need a good enough or big enough 'Why' to motivate us or inspire us to overcome inertia. Whether it's getting up from a comfy chair to take the dog out, going to a gym to do some exercise, making the phone call we have been putting off for a while or overcoming Hebbian Learning, doing that something more when we have the choice to do something less, or even nothing, requires a good enough or big enough 'Why'.

The desire to do something will usually have two drivers, which are often referred to as 'Towards and Away From Motivation'.

'Towards Motivation' means we do something because of the perceived benefit or pleasure we attach to the outcome of doing the thing we want, i.e. the pleasure we are moving towards.

'Away From Motivation' means we do something because of the perceived pain or discomfort we attach to the current situation, or the upcoming situation if we do nothing, i.e. the pain we want to move away from.

In any given situation, both will actually be present, but we often tend to have a preference for one over the other. Some people are very 'future' driven, focusing on goals and positive outcomes; others are more fear driven, doing things to escape or avoid a negative.

When I can help someone identify what their deepest motivation is for achieving something, and what type, we can focus on it and amplify it in the right way. On the surface level, it would be pointless to focus on the negative if someone is more positively driven; conversely, it would be inefficient to focus on the positive if someone responds better to the negative.

However, if I find there is *resistance* to thinking about either I will often dig into that, because we will usually find a fear, a limitation, and whenever we spot one of these and resolve it, the transformation is often more profound. We'll explore this further later on.

For now though, within each of those areas you thought about in the 'Wishlist' exercise (p. 101), there will be both towards and away from motivations, so let's go through an exercise to help identify them. These will be your 'Whys', and we can then find out whether you are still just interested in changing those areas or getting closer to being committed.

Exercise 4: A Big Enough 'Why'

Duration: 15–20 minutes
Journal Required: Yes
Buddy Required: Optional

Background

This life-coaching exercise, using Cartesian Questions, is an excellent way to help identify and clarify what your motivations for change might be in order to help create the inspiration and motivation to get on and do the things required to make those changes.

Instructions

1. On a new page in your journal, write the heading 'Health and Well-being Motivation'.
2. Underneath that, write down your *one thing that you feel needs to change in that area*, from the earlier exercise.
3. Then write out an answer for *each* of the following questions:

   Q1: What *will* happen if you *do not* resolve [this area of your life]?

   A: If I do not resolve [this area of my life] then what will happen is . . .

   Q2: What *will not* happen if you *do not* resolve this area of your life?

   A: If I do not resolve [this area of my life] then what will not happen is I won't . . .

   Q3: What *will* happen if you *do* resolve [this area of your life]?

   A: If I do resolve [this area of my life] then what will happen is . . .

   Q4: What *will not* happen if you *do* resolve this area of your life?

   A: If I do resolve [this area of my life] then what will not happen is I won't . . .

4. Repeat this process for the Career and Money motivation area and the Relationships and Intimacy motivation area, using a separate page in your journal for each.
5. Now give yourself a new motivation score out of 10 for each of the 'one thing that needs to change', where 10 = *very* and 0 = *not at all*.
6. Write your score at the bottom of each page and see if it has changed yet from your original one from the previous exercise.

Analysing Your Results

0–4 You may not particularly like the current situation but you have little or no interest or motivation towards changing it and in a way you are happy to put up with it – even though you know at some level it is probably not good for you. You may have strong fears or reservations around even thinking about change.

5–7 You have an interest in changing the situation but are not yet committed enough to do so, or have fears and reservations about the idea.

8–10 Sounds like you are ready to get on with it and just need some help to know how.

Exercise 5: Elevate Your 'Why'

Duration: 5–10 minutes
Journal Required: Yes
Buddy Required: Optional

Background

Now that we have some information to go on regarding some of the areas you would like to work on, we need to elevate the 'Why' sufficiently to enable you to actually get started and get on with it. Sometimes, however, we need to do this in stages, as below.

Instructions

1. Look at your motivation score at the bottom of *each* of the pages from the previous 'Big Enough "Why"' exercise.
2. For each one, answer the relevant question below, dependent on your score.

3. When completed, read out loud each of your three answers – one from each topic area – several times, and notice how they feel now.
4. Notice any change in your motivation score as you do.

The Questions

If you previously scored 0–4, ask yourself what would make you feel *more interested* in changing, improving or transforming that area of your life. Write down your answer underneath your motivation score in your journal, in the following format:

> *What would make me feel* **more interested** *in changing, improving or transforming this area of my life is . . .*

If you previously scored 5–7, ask yourself what would make you feel *more committed* to changing, improving or transforming that area of your life. Write down your answer underneath your motivation score in your journal, in the following format:

> *What would make me feel* **more committed** *to changing, improving or transforming this area of my life is . . .*

If you previously scored 8–10, ask yourself what sort of *help* you think you need in order to be able to get on with changing, improving or transforming that area of your life. Write down your answer underneath your motivation score in your journal, in the following format:

> *In order to be able to get on with changing, improving or transforming this area of my life now, I just need . . .*

Done it? Good. Have you read them out loud several times as instructed? Well done.

Let's move on. But don't be surprised, now, if you also suddenly find yourself willing and able to make some of those changes already.

The U-Flow Process

Whenever someone asks for my help, one of the things I am trying to figure out during the early part of our conversation is at what level do we need to operate to bring about the change they desire. Can we keep it fairly surface level? Or do we need to dig a little deeper? Will digging a little deeper suffice? Or do we need to dig *really* deep?

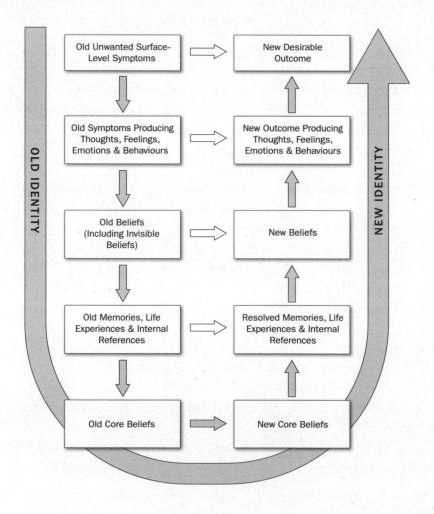

The same applies to any of us seeking to create change or transformation in our lives and the simplest way I have found to help figure it out is by what I call the U-Flow Process.

Have a look at the diagram opposite and consider some of the areas of your life that you have been thinking about changing. Can you go straight across the top, from left to right? Or do you need to dip down a level, find a crossing point lower down and come back up? If so, how far down do you need to go to find the right crossing point before you can come back up and get the transformation you desire?

If we can identify the right crossing point, we can focus our will and energy there so that the changes we require have the greatest chance to endure.

Let's go through this step by step for a moment to make sure we understand fully, and don't be surprised if ideas come to mind regarding your own situations. Feel free to note down anything you want to on a 'General Thoughts' page in your journal, but we will do a structured exercise on this in a moment, so no need to spend too much time on it just yet.

Level 1 – Surface-level Symptoms

At the top left we have our surface-level symptoms. These are the thoughts, feelings, behaviours or outcomes that have impacted our life to such an extent that they make us want to do something to alleviate or change them.

Feeling anxious? Getting angry? Biting our nails? Holding ourselves back?

Sometimes, when we realize what we have been doing and have a strong desire to do something else, we can actually reduce or stop the old way and start or increase a new way, just like that. It is a realization, followed by a decision, followed by action.

- I am no longer going to eat chocolate buttons when I walk into my kitchen, I am going to drink a glass of water instead.

- I am no longer going to drink alcohol every night during the week, I'll just have a glass of wine or beer at the weekend.
- I am no longer going to be the 'shy, uncomfortable one' when I walk into a room, I am going to be the one who puts everyone at ease by walking up to them, shaking hands and saying hello instead.
- I am no longer going to bite my nails. I am going to leave them alone so that they can grow.

These are all examples I have used myself! The general formula is:

I am no longer going to [X], I am going to [Y].

We'll need a good enough reason, or big enough 'Why', of course, to make us want to make that change, but sometimes it really can be that simple.

This is what most of us try first of all – we call it using willpower – but problems can arise if we meet internal resistance. If we have a *good enough reason*, we are *committed to the change* and our will is sufficient to overcome any resistance then we will succeed and likely establish a new way of being with new, more desirable outcomes. If not, we'll struggle, find ourselves running up that down escalator, and have to drop a level deeper.

NOTE: We can move directly from the old unwanted surface-level symptoms to the new, more desirable outcomes using our willpower, provided we are able to overcome any resistance to the change.

Level 2 – Underlying Thoughts, Feelings, Behaviours

Now, as we know, our surface-level symptoms typically only exist because of conditioning from Hebbian Learning or are adaptations and reactions to the threat response – or a combination of the two.

If we struggle to make changes at the surface-symptom level, the next step is to dip into the thoughts, feelings, emotions and behaviours that create those surface-level symptoms.

- What was I thinking or imagining that made me feel anxious about going out this evening? What was I afraid of? What did I do or want to do – either through fear or conditioning or both – to help me cope or avoid instead?
- What am I worried will happen if I do not get this work done on time? What did that make me imagine and feel? What did I want to do to compensate or cope?
- What was I thinking that made me say yes when I knew I should have said no? What was I feeling? What was I afraid of? What did I imagine it would get me?

If we can identify what the old thoughts, feelings, emotions and behaviours are that created the old surface-level symptoms, very often that in itself can begin to break the pattern or cycle, especially if we are able to talk about them with a trusted friend, colleague, family member or professional therapist.

But if we can then also create a new set of thoughts, feelings, emotions or behaviours that directly challenge the old ones – are opposites, even – and positively reinforce them by persistently focusing our conscious will and imagination *at this level*, they can filter upwards and create the new, more desirable outcomes we seek.

The general formula is:

> *What was I thinking, feeling, doing or imagining that made me do or have those surface-level symptoms in the first place?*
> *What is the opposite I would rather – or need to – think, feel, do or imagine instead so that I can create more positive desirable outcomes?*

For example:

- Instead of imagining feeling anxious and afraid, I can imagine myself having a good time, so feel better about going out.
- Instead of stressing over a work deadline, making myself feel anxious and panicky, I can stay calm and focused and just get on with doing it, so I can relax.
- Instead of saying yes when I wanted to say no, I can imagine saying no and feeling OK about it now.

Our conscious will, focused in this way, can produce powerful results, dehypnotizing us from old patterns of thoughts and consciously hypnotizing us or conditioning us to have new ideas. No mystical state needed – just a conscious focus of will.

But focusing on these new ideas to imprint them on our mind is like trying to gain access to the nightclub, and our critical faculty, gatekeeper of the mind, will be watching closely. If any of these new ideas challenge or contradict a belief we hold about ourselves or about life in this area, we know that the critical faculty will trigger the threat response and we will become divided – one part of us focusing on the new ideas, another part saying, 'Oh no you don't'.

> NOTE: We can move directly from the old thoughts, feelings, emotions and behaviours to the new, more positive thoughts, feelings, emotions and behaviours – and get the new, more desirable outcomes we desire now – provided there is acceptance from our beliefs.

If our underlying beliefs support the new ideas, great. If not, we will struggle or have inconsistent results. So we drop down another level in the U-Flow and apply the same process to our beliefs.

Level 3 – Beliefs

Beliefs are like thought factories. As we know, it is our beliefs that create the thoughts, which generate the feelings and emotions, which drive the behaviours, which create the surface-level symptoms in our lives. If we can identify the beliefs at play, and switch them for more positive ones, once again it ripples back up the U-Flow and we experience positive results.

- What must I be believing in order to have had the thoughts that make me eat foods that are 'bad' for me, instead of eating more of what I want or need to eat, in order to lose weight and feel good?
- What must I be believing that makes me screw up when I go for a promotion at work, so that I never achieve the

level of satisfaction and financial reward I know I am
capable of?
- What must I be believing to be having the thoughts that are
causing me to wake up at night and not be able to get back to
sleep?
- What must I be believing that makes me attract certain
relationships that make me feel a certain way?
- What do I need to believe instead?

The general formula is:

*What must I have been believing to have been thinking, feeling or
imagining what I was previously?*
*What do I need to believe instead, starting right now, today, that
will allow me to have a different set of thoughts, feelings, emotions
and behaviours?*

When working with a client, although we can often get change at
Level 1 and Level 2, I nearly always aim to dig down to the belief level,
at least, because that will usually be the easiest place to have a lasting
effect.

But those beliefs do not just appear for no reason, we have references
and memories and life experiences that 'prove' why we need to believe,
think and feel certain things about ourselves and our lives in that way.
If we just try to switch beliefs, when we have inner evidence to support
our contradictory beliefs, then our critical faculty may get activated and
trigger resistance – fear – the threat response, making it difficult to accept
the new beliefs.

NOTE: We can move from an old belief system to a new, more positive belief
system provided our inner referencing system – our memories and life
experiences – can provide evidence that it is OK and safe to do so.

If not, we may need to explore emotionally charged memories, impactful life experiences and any powerful internal references that have been
supporting the beliefs we have been holding on to, until now.

Level 4 – Memories and Life Experiences

As we learned from our Pyramid and Library Models of the Mind, emotionally charged life experiences can lead to emotionally charged memories, which our minds will refer to, creating emotionally charged beliefs. Once we recognize what we are believing, and the emotions those beliefs are creating, we can dig deeper into the origins and trace them back in order to not only understand the causes, but actually resolve and release them as well.

- Where did I learn to believe that I need to feel anxious at the idea of public speaking?
- Where did I learn to believe it is not safe for me to lose weight?
- What has caused me to believe I am not allowed to do what I really want to do in life?
- What have I been through that has made me feel I need to be overcontrolling of everything in order to feel safe?
- What is my mind accessing, consciously and subconsciously, that is making me believe these things?
- What is it I felt in my past that is causing the same feeling now?

In a private session, what I would usually do is help someone relax and go inward, focusing on the feelings they have been experiencing, and then let their mind slide back in time, going deeper, linking and connecting to memories and life experiences charged with similar emotion.

It is not an intellectual process, however. We are looking for the subconscious connections, the things going on beneath our awareness, so that we can bring them into our conscious awareness and deal with them. We are not necessarily trying to find buried (repressed) memories – things we have forgotten about – we are simply trying to find out what our mind is referencing that is causing us to believe what we have been believing.

This can often trigger quite painful feelings and emotions and our threat response may be on high alert at the very idea, creating resistance at first, hence the instruction to 'stay with the feeling'. But, as I have said before, on the other side of what we are afraid of feeling is release from it, if we can be brave enough to face it, acknowledge it and feel it.

In a regression therapy session like this, tapping into the emotionally charged memories would begin to dissolve any emotion attached to them, along with any limiting ideas or beliefs that had come from them, thereby reducing or eliminating their impact; but it is the old beliefs that arose from the memories that we really need to change.

This is why I would then also seek to find a way of transforming them (the memories), so that the next time our mind goes inward, looking for what to believe, it has a different reference point.

We will go through exercises on this that you can do yourself, but initially we simply need to become aware of any emotional hotspots in our memories that are making it difficult to let go of some of our limiting beliefs.

For many people, if we get this far and hit the right spot, we can usually get a pretty good transformation, fairly quickly.

There is, however, another level, one that took me many years to fully understand and appreciate, and it is what will usually bring about the greatest level of release and transformation – our core beliefs.

Level 5 – Core Beliefs

Core beliefs seem to be intrinsic to every human being in one way or another, and we will go through them in detail shortly; they are often the reason that even a deep cleansing of our past can still leave us with persistent issues.

Think back to Kate's case study. The previous hypnotherapist had done some great regression work clearing out Kate's past, the kind of thing I did myself for many years. But what we discovered, when Kate and I worked together, were core beliefs underneath all of that – and it is these that I have learned to look for and focus on in recent years.

NOTE: We can move from old, painful, emotionally charged memories to new, more positively biased inner references that give us more positive ideas, thoughts and outcomes – provided our core beliefs allow us to do so.

So when you think again of an area of life you wish to resolve, can you now see why it is perfectly understandable if you have found it difficult to do so thus far? All of these levels need to be in alignment for a change to be lasting and permanent. Conflict on any level will create resistance to change.

'Can't you just "hypnotize me" to make it all better?' people often ask. Sometimes, yes, we can just relax into that focused state of mind we call hypnosis, reduce or distract the critical faculty for a while and introduce some new, more positive ideas that serve us better. But whether we do that or dig into the causes first, it will nearly always involve a journey down one side of that U and back up the other.

Sometimes that journey is a very shallow U-shape; sometimes it is a much deeper one. As a rule of thumb, the more evidence there is of repeating patterns where we find ourselves with the same feelings but a different story, the more likely we are to have to dig deeper; the more it seems to be just a habit, with minimal emotional intensity behind it, the more we can deal with it closer to the surface.

However, so many times have people said to me, 'It's just a habit, I've already dealt with my past,' and then moments later are having huge releases as we tap into an emotional hotspot that was previously undiscovered.

One other thing to mention is that as we go through this change, there is often a notable shift in our *identity* – the way we view ourselves – but we'll cover that in more detail later, including how we can use identity in itself as a catalyst for change.

For now, let's take a closer look at core beliefs – because these form the foundation blocks of the E.S.C.A.P.E. Method.

Core Fears and Core Beliefs

After being in private practice for a few years and racking up my first few thousand hours of clients, I began reading a variety of books* that were well outside of the normal conventions.

Something just drew me to them and although I often found many of the ideas presented quite outlandish at first, a recurring theme began to appear which just would not go away. It was the idea that our life experiences were not only created by our beliefs but ultimately by just a few 'core' beliefs at that.

I didn't want to accept this at first because it actually contradicted some of what I had been taught in my analytical hypnotherapy training, and required me to step outside of my own belief system at the time.

Was it really that simple, that there were only a handful of fears which we all suffered from? Could any issue be reduced down to one of these if we probed deep enough?

I began to play around with the idea, half-heartedly looking out for these when working with clients. As the same ideas kept coming up again and again, I began to take a more serious interest. As I followed the feelings, probing deeper and deeper, time and time again I would hit one of these core ideas, and when I did there would always be a huge impact. It was as if when someone accessed, exposed and expressed one of these core ideas, there was a huge relief of pressure. When finally saying out loud that which had never been fully expressed before, a transformation would take place, often at a very deep level, with profound, life-changing results.

There was usually great initial resistance to the expressing of the ideas and very often an emotional release occurred as they did so, but afterwards there always seemed to be a sense of liberation.

* Two in particular were *The Nature of Personal Reality* by Jane Roberts and *An Act of Faith* by Jani King.

The result was that I eventually began to seek these out. I didn't want to just tell people to be positive when there was clearly inner resistance; instead, I would just keep digging – down that U-Flow – until the client eventually hit one of these core ideas by themselves. At that point I knew we were pretty deep within the client's belief system and so any change brought about at this level would have a much more profound impact than just dealing with the surface-level symptoms, or even the layers and levels in between. Rather than purely helping to solve problems, I began to seek deeper transformations.

The more familiar I became with these ideas, the more obviously they began to stand out. It was as if the invisible had suddenly become visible. I refined the process and began to refer to these as 'core fears' (in the negative version) or 'core beliefs' because they seemed to sit at the bottom of everything. A shift in these would cause a shift all the way up the other levels as well – a major dehypnotizing would occur and a lighter, freer version of the client would emerge afterwards.

To me, then, everything else became surface level, and these core fears, core beliefs became my target. It was as if I now knew where to turn the tap off, or where to find the zombie master who was giving life to the issues we were dealing with! The aim was to help the client move from the old, negative core belief to a new, more positive version.

Let's go through what these beliefs typically manifest as in turn now, along with some exercises to find out any effect they are currently having on your life. If you can master this, you will have a deep understanding of each area of struggle in your life, what is causing it and what you need do to ease or resolve it. So this is something you want to dedicate the appropriate amount of time to, as instructed in each section.

E for ENOUGHNESS

The first core belief to be aware of is around our sense of worth and value – our 'enoughness' – and this forms the E in our E.S.C.A.P.E. Method. You may be aware of this idea from other teachings but when I first read about this idea myself, back in the mid-1990s, I learned that the fundamental *fear* that goes with this first old core belief is 'I am not enough' in some way.

Old Core Belief 1: I Am Not Enough

This 'not enoughness' can play itself out in many ways. The most obvious are ideas or labels such as feeling useless, worthless, stupid, inadequate, etc., which mean we feel we are 'not [something] enough'.

- I am a bad person (not good enough)
- I am unlovable (not lovable enough)
- I am unlikeable (not likeable enough)
- I am unworthy (not worthy enough)
- I am ugly (not attractive enough)
- I am nervous (not confident enough)
- I am fat (not slim enough)
- I am short (not tall enough)
- I am small (not big enough)
- I am stupid (not clever enough)
- I am cowardly (not brave enough)
- I am boring (not interesting/funny enough)
- I am poor (not wealthy enough)
- I am unqualified (not qualified enough)
- I am a failure (not successful enough)
- I am unfit (not fit enough)
- I am [*negative label*] which means I am not [*fill in the blank*] enough . . .

And so on. Feeling guilty, bad, wrong are also expressions of this idea.

The fundamental idea is that we are lacking in some way. That *who we are* is lacking, which makes us inadequate and therefore unworthy of something good and, by inference, worthy of something not good – or bad!

If there is something we desire in life but we carry a belief around our lack of worth in that area, making us feel unworthy of it, it is highly likely we will sabotage any attempt to achieve what we want to achieve and end up feeling lacking, because as we get close to having or achieving it, our threat response will kick in and affect our behaviour as the having or achieving will be going against our beliefs.

ANY time we find ourselves saying one of these 'not enough' type of phrases, either in conversation or to ourselves as part of our self-talk, we are displaying symptoms of the 'I am not enough' core belief, and if unchallenged, will be rehypnotizing ourselves and reinforcing it.

There is a difference to be aware of though:

- I am certainly not of royal blood enough to be in line for the throne of England, and if I gave *meaning* to that (remember our 'Awareness of Meaning' exercise?), then I could begin to FEEL not enough as a person, and that would be the negative core belief playing itself out, whereas actually it just means I have a different family heritage.
- Being male, I am not female enough to play for a women's hockey team, and if I gave meaning to that, then I could begin to FEEL not enough as a person, which would then be the negative core belief playing itself out, instead of accepting that I am merely of a different gender.
- I am not tall enough to touch the moon – even if I stand on tiptoes – and if I gave meaning to that, again I could feel inadequate and not enough as a person – whereas it actually means the moon is too far away to touch.

Does that make sense?

Just because we do not have a certain quality or trait, or skill, or ability, or possession, or person in our lives, does not mean that *we* are not enough as a person. But if we attach *meaning* to that, we will *feel* not enough – and then act out a response.

Now, at first it may seem as if there are certain events in life that cause us to feel not enough, but the more I worked with these ideas, the more it seemed as if these negative core beliefs were somehow already hardwired in, to varying degrees. With these ideas hardwired in, we then found ways to experience them, or had experiences which we could hang beliefs like 'I am not enough' on to, and then experience the effect coming back to us. It was just a case of which form would they take, which characters would be involved and to what degree of intensity.

Here we are dipping into the 'nature vs nurture' debate, and what I am saying is that it seems to me that core ideas such as a lack of 'enoughness' are a part of our very nature, which then get nurtured by life to varying degrees or extremes.

The negative version of these core beliefs will create fear, which triggers the threat response, which in turn will then cause us to adapt how we think, feel and behave, accordingly.

In simple terms, if we experience low self-worth, low self-esteem or lack confidence, we may withdraw ('flight response') and shy away from anyone and anything that has the potential to cause us to feel the fear and anxiety of 'not being enough'.

Alternatively, we may try to do things ('fight response') to 'prove' that we are enough, to make up for the belief in our lack. We try to do things to appear:

- Good enough
- Lovable enough
- Likeable enough
- Worthy enough
- Attractive enough
- Confident enough
- Slim enough
- Tall enough
- Big enough
- Clever enough
- Brave enough
- Funny enough
- Interesting enough

- Wealthy enough
- Qualified enough
- Successful enough
- Fit enough

. . . and so on.

But if the drive for these comes from a belief that we are lacking, no matter what we may achieve externally in any of these areas, we will still feel a sense of lack internally, and will never quite get to feel that sense of 'enoughness' we are seeking. There may be temporary highs . . . but they will be fleeting or followed by lows, so we again end up at the bottom of the escalator, feeling inadequate or 'less than', especially if we compare ourselves to those who seem to be full of self-worth and confidence at the top.

Is it possible to change this? Absolutely, because our will and determination can go a long way, especially when applied in the right direction and in the right way. Or we can tap into emotionally charged memories and life experiences symbolizing this and release the brakes that way.

But unless we can change that core belief, it will be an ongoing battle, forever running up that down escalator, having to continually use positive self-talk or deal with the consequences.

To create deep and lasting change in this area, we need to be able to accept the positive version of this core belief – 'I Am Enough' – as a person – now – exactly as I am, and allow that to influence our more surface-level beliefs, thoughts and outcomes.

New Core Belief 1: I Am Enough

When we can begin to understand and accept the positive version – not just as an affirmation or mantra to be endlessly repeated but actually experiencing and *feeling* a sense of 'enoughness', without needing any external measure to prove it – then we can feel like a new person.

We can make different choices and say yes to things that support our 'enoughness', and no to things that don't. We can say yes to the right people, and no to the wrong; we can say yes to the good choices, and no to the lesser ones. As a result, the outer circumstances – the surface-level symptoms – begin to change into more desirable outcomes to reflect that back to us.

People who used to make us feel 'not enough' will no longer fit our version of the world, so we will either bring out different attributes in them, which reflect our new sense of self-respect, or they may move on, making way for someone new in our life.

And, ironically, the things we were striving for before can then come much more easily and effortlessly. I often say to clients and students,

'Whatever feeling drives a behaviour will usually end up creating more of the same feeling.'

If we attempt to do something from a feeling of lack and 'not enough-ness', in the end it will usually just create more of the same. If we desperately chase a new relationship from a place of feeling unloved, we will act in a way that will most likely leave us feeling rejected and unloved again! If we behave out of character, trying to make an impression on someone because we feel inferior, they are likely to see right through us and leave us feeling even more inferior than before. If we make any attempt to fix a symptom from the place of the negative core belief, we will probably just end up feeling more of the same negative belief.

But if we can find a sense of peace and strength and power and self-acceptance, for example, even within a difficult situation, the actions taken from that place – from the quiet within the storm – can lead us out of difficulty much more effectively and into more positive experiences.

The Real You is 'Enough'

The Real You *is* enough. Many people fear the opposite: 'What if I find out I am not a nice person after all?' But that is just the 'I am not enough' idea at work.

Imagine a beautiful diamond, sparkling, pristine, pure, perfect. Now imagine life throws some dirt at that diamond, and some of the dirt sticks. The diamond catches a glimpse of itself in the mirror and feels shocked – and some more dirt sticks, followed by more.

Eventually, all the diamond sees is the dirt – and so hides away, or parades itself in gaudy colours to try to make itself seem more respectable.

One day, tired of doing this and feeling knocked by life, the diamond falters and finds itself caught in a rainstorm. It feels exposed, afraid and tries to hide.

But as the rain washes away the dirt, the diamond catches a glimpse of its reflection, and slowly, gradually, remembers what it really is, and always has been. And, finally, feels peace.

So if the Real You is enough, can we just go around saying 'I am enough' a thousand times a day until it sinks in? Well, that is one way, which may work for some people, but it is unlikely to create lasting results for most of us if our critical faculty acts as gatekeeper and says, 'Who are you kidding?' Especially if we then contradict it by allowing negative thoughts and ideas to slip past unnoticed, thereby reinforcing the opposite.

This is one of the purposes of the 'Awareness of Meaning' exercises we did – so that you can begin to spot any thoughts or ideas that, if left unchallenged, will reinforce a sense of 'not enoughness', or any of the other core beliefs, which we will come on to.

We will not make much progress if we do our morning meditation or positive thinking exercise focusing on our sense of 'enoughness', believing we are solving our problem, and then spend the rest of the day undoing it.

If we are to genuinely feel our sense of innate 'enoughness', worth, value and the purpose that comes from that, we must also be willing to face the opposite – our fear – and deal with it.

As we do, however, our dear old threat response will kick in to try to prevent us from going there: 'I believe I am not enough in some way, but I don't want to feel that raw emotion, so I will do things I think will help me not feel it.'

The problem is, as we know, if we have enough emotional investment or attachment to *any* idea or belief, it *will* find a way to make itself known and turn up as events or experiences in our life that reflect it back to us. So, ultimately, we cannot just avoid it. Damn!

Or is this just a temporary 'Damn'? If life is somehow seeking to help us evolve, then each of these occasions of not feeling enough is also presenting us with an opportunity to go beyond that, to escape the limitation of the old way of thinking and instead break the pattern and begin to think, feel and experience something better. Not always easy, by any means, but very doable and very achievable – provided we are willing to be persistent and face up to a few fears.

If we can be brave enough to face up to and acknowledge the ideas we hold within ourself around lack of 'enoughness', bring them into conscious awareness for examination, expose them to the light . . . then they can dissolve, fade and disappear, leaving the positives in their place. When we feel 'enough' in any situation, we feel at peace within, and can then be more focused, more playful, more active, more restful, more effective or more whatever it is that will bring a deeper level of satisfaction and reward in that moment.

So let's do some exercises on that now.

Exercise 6: Awareness of 'Enoughness'

Duration: 10–20 minutes
Journal Required: Yes
Buddy Required: Optional

Background

Our sense of worth and value, our 'enoughness', underpins so many areas of life, so it is vital we become aware of any way in which beliefs in this area are playing a role.

This exercise is designed to assist with that and, although we are doing this in a structured way right now, you should refer back to it and use it on a regular basis if you are to make consistent and lasting progress. How often will depend on the nature and intensity of the problem you are seeking to resolve. Monthly? Weekly? Daily? Hourly? Let's do the exercises and then you can figure that out afterwards.

Instructions

Part 1

1. Go back in your journal to our very first 'Awareness of Meaning' exercise, Part 3.
2. Refer to the type of feeling or emotion note you made next to each of the people that came to mind, where P stands for positive, F (negative) now stands for Fear and M stands for a mixture of positive and fear.
3. Think of them now in terms of this 'enoughness' idea.
4. If you marked them as a P, for a positive feeling, ask yourself if any of that positive feeling is related to them helping you feel enough, or good about yourself, and in what way?
5. On a new page in your journal, labelled 'Awareness of "Enoughness"', write down the person's name and how they make you feel good or better about yourself, and look for any patterns of where you get your 'enoughness' from. Be honest! For example:

   - J. makes me feel enough because she is always complimenting me.
   - M. makes me feel enough because I can just be myself with him.
   - S. makes me feel enough because he is worse than me, which makes me feel better about myself!

Part 2

1. Again, refer to the note you made about anyone who came to mind in Part 3 of the 'Awareness of Meaning' exercise.
2. If you marked any of them as F, for a negative feeling, ask yourself if any of that feeling is related to them helping you feel not enough in some way, i.e. feeling/fearing that you are 'less than'.
3. Write down the person's name and in what way they make you feel not enough. Look for any patterns of where you get your 'not enoughness' from. For example:

- L. makes me feel not enough because I feel she is so much prettier than me.
- S. makes me feel not enough because [. . .].

Part 3

If you put M, for mixture, write down in what way they make you feel both, like this:

- [Name] makes me feel good about myself when [. . .] but not so good when [. . .].

Exercise 7: Increasing Your Sense of 'Enoughness'

Duration: 5–10 minutes
Journal Required: Possibly
Buddy Required: Optional

Background

If we rely on getting our sense of 'enoughness' from others, we will always be fearful of losing it, creating neediness. If others create a feeling of 'not enoughness' within us, we will find ourselves adapting in order to cope with that.

Every time we allow either of these two ideas to be acted out, unchallenged, we are buying into the 'I am not enough' idea, rehypnotizing ourselves that this is true and deepening the neural pathways of conditioning. However, we can interrupt it, we can slow it down, reduce it and eventually reverse it. When we hit an emotional hotspot, we can often let go of it in an instant.

Instructions

You can do the following exercise by reading and remembering it; you can make a recording using a voice note on your phone; you can have an E.S.C.A.P.E. Buddy read it to you; or do the relaxation and focus bit first of all, then open your eyes and read the ideas to yourself, closing your eyes afterwards to let them sink in.

1. Find somewhere quiet, take a few long, slow breaths, ideally breathing in through your nose and out through your mouth. If you can, breathe into your belly area first, then expand up to your chest.
2. Make the out-breath longer than the in-breath, so that it feels like a very gentle sigh of relief, as in earlier exercises.
3. Close your eyes as you breathe out, and focus on your breathing, allowing the muscles of your body to relax as you do.
4. Maintain several more of these sigh-of-relief-type breaths.
5. Pay attention to any thoughts that come up for you, but as you breathe out, imagine blowing them away and refocusing your attention on to your breath.
6. Tell your body to *relax*. (Sometimes it is easier to tell our bodies to relax than it is to tell ourselves to relax.)
7. After a few more normal breaths, let your mind focus deeper within yourself and feel around for a place deep within, away

from the normal world, beyond the thoughts and fears and
limitations of your life. Feel around inside for a feeling of deep,
deep peace, or the idea of it at the very least.

8. Take as long as you need to do this. It will get quicker and
easier each time you do.

9. Once you feel a little calmer, or have a sense of this idea of deep
peace within you, say to yourself three times:

> *The Real Me is enough, always has been and always will be, and
> does not need to prove that to anyone, in any way. If I wish to go
> and achieve things, that's fine, but my innate 'enoughness' exists
> and remains, unquestionable, whether I achieve or do not achieve.
> The Real Me does not need to seek validation from others. The
> Real Me does not need to seek 'not enoughness' or invalidation
> from others or from myself. The Real Me is enough – and therefore
> worthy and valid – now, in this moment, by the very fact that
> I exist.*

You can repeat more times if you wish, or even change the words to
something more personal to you, but it is not about the words – it is
about the *feeling* they create, and what they are helping you to reach
for. What you are reaching for is the Real You and when you can
begin to accept the validity of these statements, these words and
phrases will begin to come back to you when you need them. They
will become part of your inner self-talk. You may find it easier or more
effective to make them 'You/Your' at first, for example, 'The Real *You*
is enough . . .' etc.

Any time you can do this, wholeheartedly, you will make more
progress than you realize. Any time you can be brave enough to let go
of the idea of gaining 'enoughness' from others, and any time you can
be brave enough to let go of the need or subconscious desire to gain
'not enoughness' from others, or by negative self-talk from yourself,
you will be dehypnotizing yourself and undoing any conditioning.

Any time you authentically reach for that Real You and remind
yourself that the Real You is enough, you will be bringing that you

closer to the surface, and in so doing taking a step closer to that future you who is already there.

Although it can seem to take time to do this, any time you can you will be reducing stress and limitation in your life, so it would not be a waste of time to do this exercise several times during the day, especially when you first begin.

Here is a simpler version you can use through the day, any time you sense you are gaining either 'enoughness' or 'not enoughness' from others, or giving yourself 'not enoughness' through negative self-talk. Imagine a big red 'STOP' sign, take a deep breath and, as you breathe out, say to yourself:

> *The Real Me does not need 'enoughness' from others; the Real Me does not need 'not enoughness' from others or myself. The Real Me is enough – always has been and always will be.*

You may have to do this a number of times for it to take effect, but the first step is often just an awareness and verbalization of an idea.

Resistance

If you find this exercise difficult or experience resistance in the form of an inner voice saying, 'Yeah, but . . .', that's OK. Do not ignore it. If you can persist and *reach past it*, deeper, to the Real You, do that. If not, pay attention to the inner fear or objection and ask yourself, 'What am I afraid of here?'

In your journal, be sure to make a note of any answer, in the following format: 'I am afraid of accepting that the Real Me is enough, because . . .'

The answer will be your critical faculty talking, revealing inner resistant beliefs, and probably means this has triggered a threat response from one of your other core beliefs – which we will go through shortly – and you will need to deal with it in a similar way.

S for SAFENESS

Safeness forms the S in our E.S.C.A.P.E. Method, and as fears go, this one may be a little more obvious because, basically, if we feel unsafe then we are going to experience a degree of fear and anxiety, which is normal! But there are many ways to feel that 'the world is not a safe place for me', which is the form in which I first came across this idea.*

We can feel physically unsafe – but we can also feel unsafe or insecure financially; or in relationships; or in the workplace, for example. However we experience it, we are left feeling unable to relax and trust because we do not feel safe.

Old Core Belief 2: I Am Not Safe
(The world is not a safe place for me)

If we experience a trauma – whether as a child or adult – it will change our view on life, we will see the world differently, and that may make us feel insecure and unsafe in similar circumstances thereafter. If a beautiful mountain that we have lived by and looked up to all of our lives suddenly erupts and becomes an active, violent and unpredictable volcano, we will never quite relax in the way we had previously.

People who have been through experiences where they have been attacked physically, emotionally or sexually can often no longer feel safe in the world, especially when their trust has been broken; or where someone should have taken care of them but didn't; or they are left on their own; or they have their stability removed by a sudden change in circumstances, like parents separating or moving home. All of these can instil a feeling of insecurity and uncertainty, making us feel unsafe in the world.

What if, as a child, we experience both disruption at home and tension at school – or more extremes of those? Where does that leave us?

* In *An Act of Faith* by Jani King.

Where is our safety? Again, it will feel as if all the world is unsafe for us, and that idea may carry through into other areas as we grow up and mature, creating difficult relationships, work situations and social inter-actions, for example.

When the world no longer feels safe, our threat response can be on high alert, or we can subconsciously seek out or expect unsafe situations to arise. We may subconsciously choose or attract 'unsafe' people and circumstances, or make decisions and choices that somehow keep the unsafe cycle going. The patterns will repeat and with each repetition we will be reinforcing the fear-based ideas, rehypnotizing ourselves and reconditioning ourselves, believing we are right to do so because that is what our experience brings us.

Only when we can break the pattern, see beyond the experiences, resolve any beliefs, release any suppressed or repressed emotions and find a new way of thinking will we begin to have new experiences and trust in them.

Feeling safe in the world is also connected to our sense of worth, value and 'enoughness'. If we have poor or low self-worth we can often feel very unsure of ourselves in a variety of situations. Scenarios that are fun and relaxing to some can be extremely challenging to others, trig-gering the threat response so we would much rather just get out and get home – assuming home is a safe place – or not go there in the first place.

The basic outcome we expect as a result of this belief is that we are vulnerable to attack in some way. Feeling unsafe and vulnerable to attack can lead to long-term stress and anxiety, and have a direct impact on sleep and a whole variety of physical and emotional issues.

Many of us desperately want to make changes in our lives, knowing that the current conditions are not good for us – but we also feel unsafe making those changes, sometimes consciously or sometimes subcon-sciously, if the beliefs are more invisible.

If we have always got our sense of 'enoughness' from an external source, for example, it can seem unsafe to not have that any more, mak-ing the previous exercise on dehypnotizing lack of self-worth ('Increasing Your Sense of "Enoughness"') tricky at first.

All resistance is fear, remember, so if we feel resistance to change, it is because we feel unsafe doing so. We may need to allow ourselves to first focus on the idea that it is *safe* to allow the change, before we can focus on the change itself. Does that make sense? We will do exercises on this shortly, to clarify.

We can often project unsafe qualities on to people or situations that *are* safe. The same process of our mind perceiving something via our senses, checking inside for what we know or believe, and then having fear-based memories or imaginings kick in as a response can make us project past experiences of 'unsafeness' on to current and future situations where, actually, we can now be safe.

When we can break this old pattern of conditioned responses and behaviours and find a sense of safeness and security within ourselves, we can finally begin to feel safe in the world; we can finally begin to trust the right people – and know how to recognize them; we can find ourselves making decisions and taking actions that lead to a genuine increase in our sense of security; we can finally feel safe enough to relax, let go and be ourselves; and our life experiences can evolve to reflect that back to us.

Then, as we venture out into the world, we do so with a deeper level of safeness and security that comes from within. It doesn't mean we need to be reckless; it does mean we can have more appropriate responses to the people and events in our life, whether real and current, past and remembered, future and imagined.

The net effect is that we experience deeper levels of calmness, happiness, freedom and, ultimately, a deeper sense of peace.

New Core Belief 2: I Am Safe
(The world is a safe place for me)

The Real You is Safe

When our level of safeness is challenged, we feel vulnerable to attack and so can attack back or strike pre-emptively. But every time we attack or have an attack thought, even if directed towards another, we are actually attacking ourselves. We are attacking our beliefs around safeness and we may even be attacking our body and immune system as well. *The Real You does not need to attack. The Real You is safe.*

Remember, attack is a response to threat or danger, so if we are having attack thoughts we must, at some level, be experiencing threat, thereby believing in a lack of safeness.

Every attack thought – whether directed at ourselves or another – is ultimately an attack on ourself and our level of safeness. To view another person as less than us only shows a lack of 'enoughness' in ourselves. To attack or weaken another, physically, psychologically or emotionally is a sign of defensiveness in ourselves – we must feel weak, unsafe or vulnerable to attack to do so. How many wars have been started through a belief in a lack of 'enoughness' or lack of safeness, either physically or ideologically?

The Real You is enough and so feels no need to attack another in order to gain 'enoughness' and feel safe. The Real You is enough and so has no need to defend itself, mentally or emotionally, from another's perceived attack.

As the belief strengthens, the version of the world you experience, through choices and actions, will become a safer place to be. The Real You is not blind to real physical danger, however, should it arise, and is still able to respond to a real life-threatening situation, such as avoiding a moving car, for example. But the Real You is not looking for it, expecting it or subconsciously seeking it out.

In normal, everyday life, the Real You is – and feels – safe, deep within, and with that comes a deep sense of peace.

Exercise 8: Awareness of Safeness

Duration: 10–20 minutes
Journal Required: Yes
Buddy Required: Optional

Background

As with 'enoughness', our sense of safeness or vulnerability to attack underpins so many areas of life, and it is vital we become aware of any way in which beliefs in this area are playing a role.

Remember, the aim of this exercise is to help you raise that awareness – to make the invisible visible, the subconscious conscious – so that we can stop subconsciously reacting and instead begin to consciously create change.

Although we are doing this in a structured way right now, you should refer back to the exercise and use it on a regular basis if you are to make consistent and lasting progress. Again, how often will depend on the nature and intensity of the problem you are seeking to resolve.

Instructions

Part 1

1. Go back in your journal to our very first 'Awareness of Meaning' exercise, Part 3.
2. Refer to the type of feeling or emotion note you made next to each of the people that came to mind, where P stands for positive, F (negative) now stands for fear and M stands for a mixture of positive and fear.
3. Think of them now in terms of this safeness idea.
4. If you marked them as a P, for a positive feeling, ask yourself if any of that positive feeling is related to them helping you feel safe or increasing your level of safeness, and in what way.
5. On a new page in your journal, labelled 'Awareness of Safeness', write down the person's name and in what way they make you feel safe or safer, and look for any patterns of where you get your safeness from. Be honest! For example:

   • T. makes me feel safe because she never criticizes me and I can just be myself.
   • D. makes me feel safe because he is always there and I know he will always drop everything for me.
   • V. makes me feel safe because whenever I lose it, she has a way of making me see sense.

Part 2

1. Again refer to the notes you made about anyone who came to mind in Part 3 of the 'Awareness of Meaning' exercise.
2. If you marked any of them as F, for a negative feeling, ask yourself if any of that feeling is related to them making you feel unsafe (fear) in some way, or vulnerable to attack.
3. Write down the person's name and in what way they make you feel unsafe, and look for any patterns in the ways in which others make you feel unsafe. For example:

   - G. makes me feel unsafe because I never know whether she is going to explode at me or not.
   - H. makes me feel unsafe when he drinks and gets abusive.
   - [Name] makes me feel unsafe because/when [. . .].

Part 3

If you put M, for mixture, write down in what way they make you feel both:

   - [Name] makes me feel safe when [. . .] but not safe when [. . .].

Part 4

1. Let your mind roam freely for a while searching for any other persons or circumstances in your life causing you fear, unease or anxiety right now.
2. For each one, ask yourself, 'What am I afraid of? What do I think will happen?'
3. Write your answers in your journal as follows:

   - At the moment, when I think of [. . .] I do not feel safe because I am afraid that [. . .].

NOTE: Be sure to avoid filtering and make sure to include *everything* that you bring to mind here, even if it feels uncomfortable. Criticism and judgement are all forms of attack so be sure to include these.

Part 5

1. Repeat Part 4, but become aware of any way in which you 'attack' or make the world 'unsafe' for anyone else – which may include being physically threatening or violent, or psychologically attacking through criticism, ridicule and judgement, or even just *thinking* such attack thoughts.
2. Make a set of summary statements in a format something like this:

   - These are the ways in which I feel unsafe and vulnerable to attack from others . . .
   - These are the ways in which I attack myself . . .
   - These are the ways in which I externalize this and end up attacking others, whether physically, psychologically or imaginatively . . .

Feeling unsafe and vulnerable to attack can actually lead us on to another of the core beliefs, which we will explore in a moment, but first let's do an exercise to help us begin increasing our sense of safeness.

Exercise 9: Increasing Your Sense of Safeness

Duration: 5–10 minutes
Journal Required: Possibly
Buddy Required: Optional

Background

If we are to feel safer in the world, in our lives, in ourselves, we must feel free from all forms of attack. Otherwise the threat response will cause us to think, feel and behave in ways designed to protect us, which we may experience as annoying or debilitating surface-level symptoms.

Any time we can reduce or end ideas of attack, we are increasing our sense of safeness, which switches off the threat response, allowing us to feel calmer and more peaceful, allowing more of our Real Self to come to the surface.

Instructions

You can do the following exercise by reading and remembering it; you can make a recording using a voice note on your phone; you can have an E.S.C.A.P.E. Buddy read it to you; or do the relaxation and focus bit first of all, then open your eyes and read the ideas to yourself, closing your eyes afterwards to let them sink in.

1. Find somewhere quiet, take a few long, slow breaths, as before, relaxing your shoulders on the exhale.
2. Make the out-breath longer than the in-breath, so that it feels like a very gentle sigh of relief, as in earlier exercises.

3. Close your eyes as you breathe out and go within, allowing the muscles of your body to relax as you do.
4. Maintain the breathing for several more of these sigh-of-relief-type breaths.
5. As you do, pay attention to any thoughts that come up for you, but as you breathe out, imagine blowing them away and refocusing your attention on your breath.
6. Tell your body to *relax*.
7. After a few more normal breaths, let your mind focus deeper within yourself and feel around for a place deep within, away from the normal world, beyond the thoughts and fears and limitations of your life. Feel around inside for somewhere safe, with a feeling of deep, deep peace, or the idea of it at the very least.
8. Take as long as you need to do this. It will get quicker and easier each time you do.
9. Once you feel calmer or have a sense of this deep peace within you, say to yourself three times:

> *The Real Me is safe and secure in the world. The Real Me does not seek attack from others and the Real Me does not seek attack from myself. The Real Me is free of attack. The Real Me does not need to attack others and the Real Me does not need to attack myself. The Real Me stops any and all thoughts of attack. The Real Me is safe and secure and can relax.*

You can repeat more times if you wish, and customize the words if you prefer, but again, it is not about the words – it is about the *feeling* they create, and what they are helping you to reach for. What you are reaching for is a you – what we are calling the Real You – who feels a deep sense of peace, of safeness, where attack and defence are not required. You may find it easier or more effective to use 'You/Your' instead at first, for example, 'The Real *You* is safe . . .' etc.

Any time you can do this, even for a moment, you will begin to break the old conditioning and programming, and thereby increase your sense of safeness. Any time you allow attack thoughts to persist, unchallenged, you will be rehypnotizing and reinforcing the opposite.

Here is a simpler version you can use through the day, any time you sense you are feeling under attack or having attack thoughts yourself. Imagine a big red 'STOP' sign, take a deep breath and, as you breathe out, say to yourself:

> *The Real Me does not need attack from others; the Real Me does not need attack from myself; the Real Me does not need to attack others. The Real Me is safe and secure and can relax.*

Again, you may have to do this a number of times for it to take effect, but the first step is just awareness of the effect as you do – whether your mind can accept the ideas or whether it is resisting.

Resistance

If you sense any resistance to this idea, that is OK and perfectly normal. If you can persist and *reach past it*, deeper, to the safety of the Real You, great, do that. If not, pay attention to the inner fear or objection and ask yourself, 'What am I afraid of here?'

In your journal, be sure to make a note of any answer in the following format: 'I am afraid of accepting that the Real Me is safe because . . .'

The answer will be your critical faculty talking, revealing inner thoughts, ideas and beliefs you hold around this, and may even be triggering one or more of your other core beliefs, which we will move on to now.

C for CONTROL

The C in our E.S.C.A.P.E. Method refers to our sense of control.

'What's that like?' I will say as the umpteen thousandth client (despite everyone being a unique and individual person) describes the situation in their mind using almost identical words to the thousands before them: *'Helpless, scared, I can't control what's happening, I can't do anything about it.'* In a curious sort of way, I am always pleased when I hear this because it means we have hit a core belief and their life is about to change.

Old Core Belief 3: I Have No Control
(I am helpless, powerless, unable to influence what happens)

'I am powerless' is the form in which I originally read about this idea. Since then I have found that, although feeling powerless is the true underlying meaning, clients rarely use that phrase; 'helpless' and 'out of control' are used far more frequently.

There are so many areas in which we can feel helpless, powerless and out of control: eating, drinking, gambling, sex, work, relationships, life. And this core belief is often connected to the first two that we've explored: feeling unsafe and worthless.

If I feel helpless, powerless and have no control, I feel unsafe and vulnerable to attack or danger, and I feel useless or not good enough for not being able to do anything about it (whatever 'it' is).

Perhaps hundreds of times I have heard people describe almost an identical scene when accessing memories while relaxed in natural hypnosis. It goes something like this: 'I am sitting on the stairs. I can hear my parents arguing. They are fighting. I am scared. I don't know what's going to happen. I want to make it stop but I am too young, too little, too small. I feel so helpless and powerless, so out of control, I don't know what to do, and I feel so scared and so ashamed because I can't do anything about it.'

And this moment, with its intense emotions, focus of attention and inability to stop it or make it better, penetrates deep into the child's subconscious as 'the way life is', hypnotizing the child to then recreate the pattern again and again in a multitude of ways, through adolescence and into adulthood. Seeking out people and situations to recreate these emotions, each time feeling helpless, powerless and out of control, each time feeling afraid or ashamed as a result, the child-turned-adult finds themselves trapped in situations, trying to make changes but powerless to do so, thereby making themselves feel even worse.

Gambling addictions, alcohol addictions, eating disorders, sexual addictions, habits and any behaviour where we feel out of control and helpless to change will most likely be firing off this core belief in one way or other. Stuck in a job? Trapped in a relationship? Feeling scared on a plane, train or driving on the motorway? These are all common places where people have described feeling stuck, trapped or out of control.

If it is a fairly new feeling to us, we can probably look at more surface-level solutions; but if this feels familiar, like a repeating pattern throughout life, it may possibly track back to earlier experiences that got locked into us, thereby creating an outlet for the negative version of this core belief.

Whether intentionally stuck or trapped as in by a perpetrator in an abuse situation, or feeling stuck or trapped as a result of an accident, such as a traffic incident, broken lift or in a cupboard during a childhood game of hide and seek that goes wrong, the same level of helplessness or lack of control over a situation can create panic at first and set up an emotionally charged belief.

If the stuck or trapped feeling is persistent in life, the lack of control and helplessness can also lead to a 'what's the point?' feeling.

From my experience, this stuck, helpless, powerless, out-of-control belief lies at the bottom of many cases of depression. If we cannot see a way out of where we are and so have no potential for a *positive, viable future* to look forward to – and feel powerless to do anything about it – eventually we just cave in, feel 'what's the point?', collapse psychologically and experience depression.

The medical approach to counteract this is to provide medication to boost the happy chemicals in our brain, and although I have thankfully seen many people's lives saved by this, it is obviously only a one-dimensional solution. Ideally, it should be used as a short-term measure while the underlying causes are worked out and resolved.

In any situation where we feel helpless, powerless and out of control, we need to become aware of the thoughts, feelings or beliefs that are causing us to feel that way and resolve any conflicts.

Once we can recognize the ideas that are causing it, we can discover that we are actually more powerful and more in control than we realize, and so the fear or depression lifts as the core fears (i.e. the negative versions) become core beliefs (the positive ones).

Coming out of this, clients will often say they feel stronger, more powerful and back in control.

New Core Belief 3: I Am Strong, Powerful and In Control

CASE STUDY: *Lifting Dominic's Depression*

Very recently I was chatting to a young man named Dominic who had been suffering with anxiety and depression for several months. He had been off work and become very unresponsive to family and friends, wanting to hide himself away.

We spoke for about an hour altogether and in our initial conversation I was wondering which of the core fears would be at play here, responsible for creating this. By asking the kind of questions I have been teaching you to ask yourself in the exercises we have done so far, pretty quickly it became apparent that what he was actually suffering from was a mixture of *fear* and *grief.*

An aunt he was very close to had died some years earlier and this had been a considerable loss to him, one that he had been unable to process and resolve, as far as I could tell. When a second aunt was recently diagnosed with a similar illness, it triggered all the old feelings – and he was anticipating having to go through the loss all over again.

He felt scared, helpless, powerless and out of control of the whole situation. He could only imagine a bleak future in which he lost another close relative. It all became too much and he withdrew; unable to fully verbalize what was going on inside and unable to conceive of a positive, viable future for himself, he became depressed.

The first thing I did was help him to resolve his grief over the aunt that had died. Without that, I would struggle to deal with the current situation because to me they were inextricably linked.

I asked him to relax using the simple breathing methods mentioned earlier and asked that his mind go inward, following the feelings we had just been talking about.

His mind took him back to the events around the first aunt, so I had him verbalize – while his eyes were closed, in the natural hypnosis 'access state' – and express everything that he had been unable to thus far, not describing it as if it were in the past, but using the present tense, *as if he were there once again.*

He described everything that was happening, but we were still not getting the response I needed for his beliefs to shift. So I took him through an exercise I use a lot when there has been any kind of grief.

I had him imagine a beautiful, enchanted glade where he was safe and protected, and into that glade walked the aunt who had died, so that he could have a chance to say anything that had not yet been said.

My aim here was twofold. One, I wanted to have him express anything that he had been thus far unable to, including thanks and appreciation to the aunt for being there for him and helping him feel loved and so on. And two, I wanted to help him build a connection with the aunt who had died, so that he could still feel comfort from her presence even though she was no longer physically with us.

The session went well, with lots of release of emotion, and creating an idea of continued connection addressed a core belief – safeness. With the increased sense of safeness, instead of feeling stuck, trapped and scared, he now felt lighter, freer, back in control of his feelings and emotions, more able to relax and get on with life.

I also taught him the 'in through the nose/out through the mouth' breathing technique that he could use any time he needed to feel calm and relaxed.

I received a note from his mother a few days later saying that there had been an almost immediate shift in him: he had joined the family to watch TV together and had spoken with his brother, whom there had been some tension with until that point.

Interestingly, a couple of weeks later he experienced a sudden dip because his girlfriend now had a major health scare, triggering the similar ideas all over again, although this time the effect was not quite so intense. See how the patterns try to repeat?

His girlfriend's issue turned out to be a false alarm and when I caught up with him briefly about a month after the initial session he was back at work, back in routine, going to the gym, feeling positive and just getting on with life. Acknowledging the real fear in the session we did, releasing the trapped emotion and using the breathing technique to help condition a new response afterwards, meant the depression had lifted. He looked like a completely different person!

This was relatively simple to resolve by asking the right questions to elicit what was really happening – i.e. what the real fear was – releasing any suppressed or repressed emotion and then using the power of his own mind and imagination to create a more positive inner referencing system.

As he became free of the past, less scared of the future and able to see how he had more control over himself and his feelings than he realized, he felt back in control, more secure, and his confidence returned. Can you see how the beliefs link together?

Control led to security (safeness), which led to self-confidence ('enoughness').

NOTE: When we can feel in control without needing to be controlling, we can feel strong, powerful and able to impact change. The world feels safer and our self-esteem and self-worth ('enoughness') gets a boost as well as we begin to feel better about ourselves.

The Real You is Powerful and In Control

The Real You is more powerful than you realize. The Real You, unleashed, is strong, powerful and in control of its thoughts, feelings and emotions, able to respond and adapt to life's twists and turns in incredibly invent-ive and creative ways.

But, like Superman when faced with Kryptonite, we can feel stripped of our power if we accept ideas and limitations that cause us to feel unable to wield that power, leaving us feeling powerless, weak, out of control, stuck, trapped and helpless, even though we may not be.

This can happen to most of us at times – when faced with difficult chal-lenges we have perhaps not encountered before or cannot find immediate solutions to – until we gather ourselves and find a way forward.

But if, especially in our younger, more formative years, life hypno-tizes us to believe that *this is the way life is*, feeling this way can become a default response to situations where we probably do not need to feel this way, thereby causing us to feel and believe even more that feeling powerless is a way of life and happens all the time.

One of the most common reasons I have come across that causes people to feel this is that they have given inappropriate meaning to events in their lives.

Children who witness parents fighting or going through divorce often feel responsible yet powerless to do anything about it. This leads them to take on two false ideas: the first is that it was somehow their fault, and the second is that there was something they could or should have done, but didn't. When – at the childhood belief level – they realize it was not their fault and they were not supposed or expected to do anything about it because it was not their issue to resolve, a huge sense of relief often comes flooding in with an intense release of emotion pouring out.

'It's not your fault' is one of the most powerful realizations you can have if you have been blaming yourself, consciously or subconsciously, for things that were actually not your fault and were out of your control.

Many victims of sexual abuse, or any kind of abuse, are often left feel-ing it was their fault and somehow blame themselves for not being able to say 'no' or 'stop'. What actually happens in many of these cases is that the threat response kicks in as 'freeze' or 'fawn'. They cannot fight the abuser, they cannot get away, so they freeze until their ordeal is over or become subordinate and 'allow' it to happen.

Remember, this is a subconscious, automatic survival process that kicks in, not a conscious decision. Yet many people are left feeling two levels of guilt and shame afterwards – one level for what just happened and another level for not preventing or stopping it from happening – and we must release both of these if we are to be free.

Very often this happens at ages when the critical faculty is not fully formed enough to logically dispel these ideas, so they enter the night-club and become part of the door policy, inviting more of the same in, unchallenged.

As a result, people who have been through such abusive experiences grow up feeling they do not even have a right to say 'no'; experiences that make them feel this way begin to feel normal and, again, they sub-consciously seek them out, feeling powerless and out of control in the situations and powerless and out of control in their ability to do any-thing about it.

Whatever situation you find yourself in, the Real You is there within, strong, powerful, resourceful and able to find solutions where solutions are to be found, or to let go of responsibility for seeking them when they are not.

When you peel away the fears and limitations that life has thrown at you, you discover that you are all those things, and yet with no need or desire to be controlling.

Let's do some exercises on this now.

Exercise 10: Awareness of Control

Duration: 10–20 minutes
Journal Required: Yes
Buddy Required: Optional

Background

When we feel strong, powerful and in control, we generally feel good. When we feel weak, powerless and out of control, our threat response kicks in, possibly triggering an anger outburst or, if sustained, usually the opposite, causing us to become withdrawn or stuck, behave subordinately or even collapse into depression. Either way, we feel bad. If we are at the bottom of that escalator, we can become scared to get back on again or not know how to even try.

If we can become aware of where this is happening, and recognize it as such, we can then begin to do something about it.

Instructions

Part 1

1. As we have done before, go back in your journal to our very first 'Awareness of Meaning' exercise, Part 3.
2. Referring to the positive, negative, neutral or mixed responses to the people who came to mind, feel around for any way in which this idea of 'control' is playing out.
3. Pay attention to anyone who is making you feel weak, powerless and out of control.
4. Pay attention to any way in which you are doing the same to others – whether by thought or deed.
5. On a new page in your journal, labelled 'Awareness of Control', write down the person's name and in what way you recognize that control beliefs are having an influence. Be honest! For example:

   - A. makes me feel weak because I do not stand up for myself.
   - M. makes me feel powerful because he always does what I say and I can control him.
   - G. makes me feel trapped because I want to be myself but feel I have to be how he wants me to be.
   - Z. makes me feel strong, powerful and in control because she is there when I need her, but allows me to be independent when I do not.

Remember, this is about raising awareness of the ways in which these ideas are playing out in your life. It is OK to be absolutely and completely honest with yourself and free of judgement. On the other side of facing up to things is the liberation of never having to face up to them again.

Part 2

1. Close your eyes and think about this idea of feeling stuck, trapped, helpless, powerless or out of control.
2. Search around inside for any familiarity of this feeling and let your mind link and connect to times, scenes and situations where you are currently experiencing this or have done in the past.
3. Make a note in your journal as to whether you are the one feeling stuck, weak, helpless, powerless or out of control . . . or whether you are trying to gain that for yourself by attempting to control, dominate or weaken another.
4. For each one, ask yourself, 'What am I afraid of? What do I think will happen if I don't do this?'
5. Write your answers in your journal as follows but feel free to adjust the wording a little if it helps:

   - In [this situation] where I feel [helpless, powerless or out of control], I do this so that [. . .] and I am scared to change because [. . .].
   - In [this situation] where I am being [controlling, dominating, overbearing], I do this so that [. . .] and I am scared to stop doing this because [. . .].

NOTE: Be sure to avoid filtering and include everything, even if it feels uncomfortable.

Feeling weak, powerless and out of control can actually lead us on to another of the core beliefs, which we will explore in a moment, but first let's do an exercise to help us begin increasing our sense of power and control, without needing to be controlling.

Exercise 11: Increasing Your Sense of Inner Strength, Power and Control

Duration: 5–10 minutes
Journal Required: Possibly
Buddy Required: Optional

Background

When we feel weak, powerless and out of control, our threat response will activate, causing us to behave in a defensive, protective or coping way. It may cause us to perpetuate the weakness and powerlessness; or it may seek to regain control over it by creating it in others, giving us a temporary illusion of strength and power. Either way, ultimately, we are in defensive mode rather than relaxed, happy and free.

Instructions

As with previous similar exercises, you can do the following exercise by reading and remembering it; by making a recording using a voice note on your phone; by having an E.S.C.A.P.E. Buddy read it to you; or do the relaxation and focus bit first of all, then open your eyes and read the ideas to yourself, closing your eyes afterwards to let them sink in.

1. Find somewhere quiet, take a few long, slow breaths, as before, relaxing your shoulders on the exhale.
2. Make the out-breath longer than the in-breath, so that it feels like a very gentle sigh of relief, as in earlier exercises.
3. Close your eyes as you breathe out and go within, allowing the muscles of your body to relax as you do.

4. Maintain the breathing for several more of these sigh-of-relief-type breaths.

5. As you do, pay attention to any thoughts that come up for you, but as you breathe out, imagine blowing them away and refocusing your attention on your breath.

6. Tell your body to *relax*.

7. After a few more normal breaths, let your mind focus deeper within yourself and feel around for a place deep within, away from the normal world, beyond the thoughts and fears and limitations of your life. Feel around inside for somewhere safe, with a feeling of deep, deep peace, or the idea of it at the very least.

8. Take as long as you need to do this. It will get quicker and easier each time you do.

9. Once you feel calmer or have a sense of this deep peace within you, say to yourself three times:

> *The Real Me does not need to feel helpless, powerless and out of control. The Real Me is strong, powerful and in control.*
>
> *The Real Me does not need to control others to make myself feel better or safer. The Real Me allows others to feel strong, powerful and comfortably in control of themselves.*
>
> *The Real Me is in control of myself, yet without being overcontrolling. The Real Me does not need to control life. The Real Me is strong enough and powerful enough to flow with what happens, adapting and evolving where needed in order to survive and thrive.*

You can repeat this more times if you wish, and amend the words to suit, but again, it is not about the specific words – it is about the *feeling* they create and the Real You that they are helping you to reach for.

Any time you can do this, wholeheartedly, you will make more progress than you realize. Any time you can be brave enough to let go of the idea of gaining control by controlling others, and any time you can be brave enough to let go of the need or subconscious desire to seek feeling out of control, you will be dehypnotizing yourself and undoing any conditioning.

Whenever you authentically reach for that Real You and remind yourself that the Real You is strong, powerful and in control, you will be bringing that you closer to the surface and in so doing taking a step closer to that future you who is already there.

You will be reducing stress and limitation in your life, so it would not be a waste of time to do this exercise several times each day, especially when you first begin.

Here is a simpler version you can use through the day, any time you sense you are feeling helpless, powerless and out of control, or about to try to make another feel that way. Imagine a big red 'STOP' sign, take a deep breath and, as you breathe out, say to yourself:

> *The Real Me does not need to control or be controlled. The Real Me is strong enough and powerful enough to feel comfortably in control of myself, able to adapt to whatever happens, and allow others to be in control of themselves, and that is OK.*

Resistance

If you find this exercise difficult or experience resistance, again that is OK. If you can persist and *reach past it*, deeper, to that sense of deep peace, do that. If not, pay attention to the resistance which, as you know, is a fear, and see if you can identify it. Ask yourself, 'What am I afraid of here?'

In your journal, be sure to make a note of any answer in the following format: 'I am afraid of accepting that the Real Me is strong, powerful and in control because . . .'

The answer will reveal inner beliefs, and probably means this idea has triggered a threat response from one of your other core fears, which we will need to deal with in a similar way.

A for ACCEPTANCE

Acceptance forms the A in our E.S.C.A.P.E. Method and I have to admit this one has been a bit of a challenge for me personally. Put up for adoption at ten days old, I developed the same symptoms that so many others who have been through similar experiences do: an inbuilt sense of low self-worth, anxiety and feeling different, like an outsider, separate, disconnected, not fitting in, not accepted, not having a place in the world, especially as I grew older. The Groucho Marx quote, 'I don't want to belong to any club that would have me as a member,' always seemed to ring very true for me.

Old Core Belief 4: I Am Not Accepted
(I do not fit in, I do not belong)

One of the reasons why I was struggling so much at that time on the train platform when the guy at the end jumped was because I was feeling torn apart inside owing to this belief. I had a beautiful young family who loved me dearly, yet 'I don't want to belong to any club – family – or relationship – that would have me as a member' seemed to be an idea that kept sabotaging my happiness.

I would swing from feeling desperately trapped and out of control within the family setting to liberated and free when out of it . . . but desperately lonely . . . and wanting back in!

'Should I stay or should I go?' sang The Clash, and I was constantly torn apart inside with this conflict, knowing it was complete madness to leave – but it was causing me a whole load of angst to stay. Aaagh!

It felt as if I somehow didn't deserve to be in this lovely, loving environment, and being there would actually trigger the threat response as a result – what I felt I *deserved* was *non-acceptance*, judgement, rejection, separation, isolation, exclusion, disconnection – and I have often been drawn to people who didn't want me, while trying to reject those who did.

Many people can experience this as a one-off in certain times of stress, but for some of us this idea can become a repeating pattern through life.

There are many forms of the 'I am not accepted' idea. Things can suddenly happen in life to make us feel different and that others will no longer accept us, things like family separations, bullying at school, physical, emotional or sexual abuse that goes unnoticed and unresolved. The general feeling is, 'There is something different or wrong about me, which means I can no longer be included. Instead, I am now separate from everyone else; I am over here and everyone else is over there, and that is how it must stay.'

Sometimes, because of other beliefs, it can seem scary to reconnect or even try to belong and fit in, so it feels safer to be separate and not fitting in. But although we may feel safe, there is loneliness as well, creating a deep desire for reconnection, even if it is consciously suppressed or repressed.

The inner conflict is often 'I want to fit in, belong and connect but I am afraid of what will happen if I do.'

Very often we rationalize it and turn it into a strength. Most of my life I have 'prided' myself on my fierce independence, my ability to cope, to manage on my own, to not need help, with an absolute, bloody-minded determination to fight back and 'prove' I am OK, believing that being outside the norm was the ideal way, even feeling panicky at the thought of being 'normal'.

All of this can and does serve a purpose at times, and can enable us to innovate, and see things differently, using that fight-response energy to drive us to keep going and get things done, long after others would have quit.

I used to get quite emotional watching the Apple advert from 1997, the one that begins . . .

Here's to the crazy ones, the misfits, the rebels, the troublemakers, the round pegs in the square holes . . . the ones who see things differently – they're not fond of rules . . .

Those first couple of lines especially gave me a sense of belonging, acceptance and even validation. Not fitting in, questioning rules and being able to see things differently are all very familiar feelings that in a way have helped me, though by and large I've been quite a well-behaved rebel because I was also scared of authority!

But it is quite a stressful way to live too. The highs see you achieve great things; the lows see you curled up in a ball, hiding from the world, having to pull it all together again for the next 'performance'. A performance may be on stage entertaining a vast crowd; it may be on the sporting field, pushing yourself to the limits; it may be running a business, leading a group or as 'simple' as attending a family gathering, full of people who love and support you (or any kind of gathering where technically there is no reason to feel afraid), and yet feeling like we don't fit in. While others are relaxing and having fun we are internally battling the threat response, wanting to connect but also to run away at the same time.

When I was first introduced to this idea it was all about connection, but I found that clients would tend to use words like 'acceptance', 'inclusion', 'belonging', 'fitting in', 'having a place in the world', and so I adapted it to suit my own experience.

There has been much written about us being social creatures who need love and acceptance to survive and thrive, but the main purpose here is just to make you aware of the 'I am not accepted' belief in case it has been invisibly playing itself out in your life, projecting itself on to any number of situations or circumstances.

What's equally important is to recognize the flip version of this belief too: when we seek to separate or exclude others, judging them for being different to us. It's a rabbit hole of a topic, but any time we judge others or exclude them or try to make ourselves feel better by looking down on others, we are really just displaying signs of our own fear of exclusion and isolation.

Back in the 1990s, when I was performing with a club punk rock band (more on this later) called Superblonde, I remember a girl coming up to me in the early hours of the morning at a particular gig we had just done in the heart of London's Soho. She placed her hands on either side of my face and looked me straight in the eyes, saying, 'Us freaks, us weirdos, have to stick together.' While part of me felt the 'Yeah, right on, rock 'n' roll' thrill and adventure, inside I suddenly felt the little boy in me want to hide and run away at the idea of being identified as such. How had it got to this, so far away from what, for me, had been the safe and loving environment of home?

Many people in that club were just having a good night out – others, like me, were desperately trying to find a tribe to belong to. On the surface I had found a place to fit in and belong, and although there were lots of fun and amazing times to be had, much of it was fuelled by a destructive angst, which eventually forced me to crash – again. The Real Me didn't belong there either, *in that way*, so where the hell did I belong? Not belonging can be a scary and lonely place.

However, when we *can* finally feel accepted – which is really about acceptance of ourselves – we discover our true place in the world and feel like at last we belong and fit in without the need to change our true selves, justify it or judge others for not being like us. We can accept ourselves for who we are and we can accept others for who they are.

We feel less need to have to adapt ourselves in order to be accepted and acceptable, and so less need to have to control things as we feel safer and more secure within ourselves and the world. This goes hand in hand with a greater sense of self-worth and self-esteem as we recognize our intrinsic 'enoughness'.

New Core Belief 4: I Am Accepted
(I belong, I have a place, I fit in, exactly as I am)

There are so many areas in which this idea of judgement and non-acceptance of ourselves and others can apply – culture, nationality, religion and skin colour, to name a few, right the way down to cliques in the playground or office politics. But one that causes a lot of fear and judgement, and can be a challenge for many, especially in our adolescent years and onwards, is the area of sexual orientation.

Take Sebastian, for example.

CASE STUDY: *Sebastian's Liberation*

When Sebastian first contacted me he had just come out of many years of psychotherapy in which he had found enormous benefit with regards to processing his rather challenging family background. Yet he was still unhappy and struggling with the sexual side of his life. He described himself as being solo-sexual but attracted to men. I understood him to mean that, although he found men attractive, he didn't actually want sex with them – he preferred that by himself. Indeed, Sebastian described to me how his solo sex sessions were closer to a tantric art form, an expression of self-love, '. . . an arena for profound, even spiritual experiencing'.

But the psychotherapist had reinforced an idea that there was actually something wrong with him, namely that he was probably just repressing homosexuality. The well-meaning psychotherapist had encouraged Sebastian to face up to his 'true nature' – that is as perceived by the psychotherapist – and seek out other men for a relationship. But each time he did this, Sebastian felt he was not being truthful to himself, leading to dissatisfaction and unhappiness.

When he had finished telling me his story, at our first meeting, a part of me was looking for the clever, psychotherapeutic answer that would explain it all and what we needed to do to fix him. But what I really, genuinely felt was, 'What's the actual problem?'

So I said something like, 'I don't see what the problem is. You find men attractive to look at, but prefer to have sexual experiences by yourself, during which time you actually often achieve a much deeper sense of connection than many couples do during sex. You have good friends, both male and female, you are not doing anyone any harm, and your sexual life is actually giving you a great deal of pleasure. What's the problem?'

It just seemed common sense to me, but to Sebastian this approach was life-changing. He had felt different, not fitting in, not acceptable, wrong in some way, but my simple acceptance seemed to have a profound effect. He later wrote to me that this acceptance had given him the support he needed to 'reclaim myself . . . for the first time . . . I was able to "show myself" completely and honestly and not strive to be something I'm not. It was cathartic, deeply therapeutic, deeply healing.'

My very matter-of-fact, but completely genuine acceptance of Sebastian had allowed him to accept himself, and he has since found a great sense of connection with others around the world with similar sexual preferences and orientation.

The Real You is Acceptable and Accepted

If we fear we are lacking in some way, not good enough, different, we can feel unsafe being ourselves and so have to adapt in order to survive. Many of us do this in certain situations – at work, for example, with the 'fake it till you make it' idea – but for many others it becomes a way of life and we have to adapt who we are and how we behave in virtually every situation. Which becomes exhausting.

The Real You is acceptable, exactly as you are. The Real You can adapt as you swap roles, from parent to employee, from business owner to best friend, from teammate to significant other, and more, but does not need to adapt who you are in each of these situations – just a different expression of who you are.

Any time we pass judgement on ourselves, we are reinforcing the 'I am not accepted' idea, usually because we feel unacceptable. This is not quite the same as 'not enough' – 'not enough' is personal to us, whereas 'not accepted' is how we relate to others.

The Real You does not need to judge yourself for who you are. There are times where we may need to be discerning – 'The way I behaved yesterday was inappropriate, I won't do that again' – but we do not need to judge and outcast ourselves for it. As mentioned earlier, you will never see a lion complaining and beating itself up because it missed its prey, and you will never see a lion cast out from the pride for doing so. It accepts itself as it is, and is accepted. But you will see a lion change tactics to avoid it happening again, learning and evolving rather than blaming.

The Real You does not need to judge or blame others and deem them 'unacceptable' either. This does not mean we need to be friends with or like everybody, or condone everything that people do – but it does mean we can acknowledge their differences and accept them for who they are and then make our decisions based on logical, rational thinking, instead of fear-based reactive thinking.

Every time we pass judgement on another, we are actually passing judgement on ourselves. We only ever *need* to pass judgement if we are somehow afraid in some way or seeking to raise ourselves up by doing so. And by the way, to truly judge something we need to know all the information from all the angles and all the perspectives. What most of us do is form an opinion based on our beliefs and expectations – which, as we know, are highly questionable in their validity as being the absolute truth because we have all been hypnotized in so many ways.

We can form an opinion, but we cannot truly judge. Many times when we feel different, unaccepted, unwanted, with no sense of place or purpose, not belonging to a particular group nor the world as a whole, it is because we hold a fear-based opinion, based on our limited interpretation of the information available, through the filter of our beliefs. However, because of the powerful and automatic nature of the threat response, it can *feel* real, and so our logic is left trying to reason with that cornered animal within us, seeking to fight or escape. It is easier to react to that than it is to sit with the feeling and ride it out long enough to dissolve the cause and break the conditioning.

When you can accept that the Real You is acceptable and can be accepted, you will stop judging others, you will stop judging yourself, and instead find a sense of peace with yourself and the world.

Exercise 12: Awareness of Acceptance

Duration: 10–20 minutes
Journal Required: Yes
Buddy Required: Optional

Background

When we feel accepted, we feel stronger, more powerful and more comfortably in control; we feel safer, better about ourselves, and as such can relax and be ourselves more, wherever we are and whoever we are with. An awareness of when we are feeling this and when we are not can help us to resolve any issues where this may be playing out in our life.

Instructions

Part 1

1. As we have done before, go back in your journal to our very first 'Awareness of Meaning' exercise, Part 3.
2. Referring to the positive, negative, neutral or mixed responses to the people who came to mind, feel around for any way in which this idea of 'acceptance' is playing out.
3. Pay attention to anyone with whom you feel completely accepted and can be yourself.
4. Pay attention to anyone who, either deliberately or unknowingly, causes you to feel unaccepted or that you do not belong.

5. Pay attention to any way in which you are being judgemental of others, deeming them unacceptable, wrong and therefore worthy of exclusion.

6. On a new page in your journal, labelled 'Awareness of Acceptance', write down the person's name and in what way you recognize the 'acceptance' beliefs having an influence. Be honest! For example:

   - S. makes me feel accepted because I can be myself and know that is OK.
   - J. makes me feel accepted, but inwardly I feel not good enough and so do not feel accepted or acceptable.
   - R. is so different to me, I just do not agree with the way she lives her life and the things she does. It is completely unacceptable.

Part 2

1. Close your eyes and think about this idea of feeling that you do not fit in, do not belong, are different, separate, rejected, disconnected even.

2. Feel around inside for any familiarity of this feeling and let your mind link and connect to times, scenes and situations where you are currently experiencing this or have done in the past.

3. Make a note in your journal as to what comes to mind and in what way it is related to this idea. Are you the one feeling rejected or outcast? Or are you the one doing the rejecting or casting out?

4. For each one, ask yourself, 'What am I afraid of? Why am I doing this? What is it helping me achieve?'

5. Write your answers in your journal as follows, but feel free to adjust the wording a little if it helps:

   - In [this situation] I am/was behaving this way because I am/was afraid that [. . .].

- I have been/was thinking that it will/would help me achieve [. . .].

For example:

- I have been avoiding taking part in the group activity because I am afraid of being laughed at. I am afraid that everyone will see through my facade and expose the worthless person I really am.
- By not taking part, or by judging them in my mind, it has helped me to feel safer and more righteous. But, actually, kind of lonely too as I feel separated from everybody.

Being honest with ourselves is vital. If we are resistant to the truth because we are ashamed or afraid to admit it, even to ourselves, we remain stuck in the threat response mode, and nothing changes. When we are honest, the subconscious becomes conscious and we can go to work on it, including using some of the exercises coming up later.

Part 3

1. Consider again this idea of judgement and non-acceptance, and let your mind expand to other people, situations and events in your life.
2. In your journal, make a note of any judgements you hold against yourself that may be possible causes for *why* you feel you are different or not accepted or don't fit in or don't belong or are not connected. List in as many areas as come to mind.

   - I am different to everyone else because . . .
   - People will not accept me here because . . .
   - I do not really belong because . . .

3. Now make a note of any judgements you hold against *others*, not accepting them as they are, wanting to reject them or change them, including any secret prejudices you may hold.

- I do not like this group of people because . . .
- I find it difficult to accept this person because . . .
- I do not want to accept these types of people because . . .
- I think these people are wrong because . . .

4. Go through your lists in 2) and 3) and identify which core beliefs thus far – lack of 'enoughness', safeness or control – each of your 'judgements' relates to. You'll need to be very honest with yourself and pay attention to the emotions you feel, including any subtle (or not so subtle) threat it is creating in you.

5. Make a summary note in your journal of anything that comes to mind, however strange or bizarre it may be. Again, these will be your beliefs being pushed to the surface, a way of making the invisible visible, the subconscious conscious. For example:

- I have been believing I didn't fit in and people wouldn't want me because I wasn't [X] enough.
- I have been unaccepting of [Y] because they make me feel [Z].
- I have been judgemental against [X] because I have been believing [Y], which was making me feel [Z].

NOTE: Any time you find yourself being judgey or non-accepting towards some-one else, take a look at your own life for a moment and feel around for any areas that you would not like exposed to others. If you judge others as unacceptable, you judge yourself in the same way; only when you can accept others for who they are can you truly accept yourself.

Feeling a sense of disconnection, separation, lack of acceptance, not belonging, not fitting in and general fear in this area, whether against ourselves or others, can actually lead us on to another of the core beliefs, which we will explore in a moment. Let's first do an exercise to help us begin increasing our sense of acceptance, of both ourselves and others.

Exercise 13: Increasing Your Sense of Acceptance

Duration: 5–10 minutes
Journal Required: Optional
Buddy Required: Optional

Background

Any time we feel unaccepted, are not accepting of ourselves or are not accepting of others, we are in threat mode. These ideas, unchallenged, will simply reinforce any existing conditioning and perpetuate the problem. When we can eliminate this from our life, we can feel at peace with ourselves, at peace with the world around us and feel we have a place and belong in it – and that's OK.

Instructions

As with previous similar exercises, you can do the following exercise by reading and remembering it; by making a recording using a voice note on your phone; by having an E.S.C.A.P.E. Buddy read it to you; or do the relaxation and focus bit first of all, then open your eyes and read the ideas to yourself, closing your eyes afterwards to let them sink in.

1. Find somewhere quiet, take a few long, slow breaths, as before, relaxing your shoulders on the exhale.
2. Make the out-breath longer than the in-breath, so that it feels like a very gentle sigh of relief, as in earlier exercises.
3. Close your eyes as you breathe out and go within, allowing the muscles of your body to relax as you do.

4. Maintain the breathing for several more of these sigh-of-relief-type breaths.

5. As you do, pay attention to any thoughts that come up for you, but as you breathe out, imagine blowing them away and refocusing your attention on your breath.

6. Tell your body to *relax*.

7. After a few more normal breaths, let your mind focus deeper within yourself and feel around for a place deep within, away from the normal world, beyond the thoughts and fears and limitations of your life. Feel around inside for somewhere safe, with a feeling of deep, deep peace, or the idea of it at the very least.

8. Take as long as you need to do this. It will get quicker and easier each time you do.

9. Once you feel calmer or have a sense of this deep peace within you, say to yourself three times:

> *The Real Me is acceptable and can feel accepted, exactly as I am. The Real Me can fit in and belong, exactly as I am. The Real Me does not need to judge, reject or exclude others. The Real Me accepts others as they are, allowing them to be different, thereby releasing me from judgement of my own differences.*

You can repeat more times if you wish, and amend the wording to make it more personal, but as stated before, it is not about the words – it is about the *feeling* they create and what they are helping you to reach for. What you are reaching for is a sense of total self-acceptance because this is what the Real You has and feels.

Any time you can do this, wholeheartedly, you will make more progress than you realize. Any time you can be brave enough to let go of the idea of not feeling accepted and any time you can be brave enough to let go of the need or subconscious desire to seek out feeling not accepted, you will be dehypnotizing yourself and undoing any conditioning.

Any time you authentically end judgement of yourself or another and instead reach for the Real You who is free from all that, and remind yourself that the Real You is completely acceptable, you will be bringing that you closer to the surface and, in so doing, taking a step closer to that future you who is already there.

Here is a simpler version you can use through the day, any time you sense you are feeling judged or not accepted, any time you feel you are judging and not accepting yourself and any time you are judging and not accepting another. Imagine a big red 'STOP' sign, take a deep breath and, as you breathe out, say to yourself:

The Real Me does not need to judge or feel judged. The Real Me accepts myself and is accepting of others.

Resistance

If you find this exercise difficult or experience resistance, again that is OK. If you can persist and *reach past it*, deeper, to that sense of deep peace, do that. If not, pay attention to the resistance which, as you know, is a fear, and see if you can identify it. Ask yourself: 'What am I afraid of here about accepting myself or allowing myself to feel accepted? What am I afraid will happen if I do? What am I afraid of about accepting others?'

In your journal, be sure to make a note of any answer, in the following format: 'I am afraid of accepting that the Real Me is acceptable, and allowing myself to feel accepted because . . .' 'I am afraid of accepting [others] because . . .'

The answers may reveal conflicting beliefs, possibly relating to the fifth and final core belief we need to become aware of now.

P for PLEASURE

The fifth letter, P, in our E.S.C.A.P.E. Method, stands for Pleasure. The *Oxford English Dictionary* defines pleasure as, 'A feeling of happy satisfaction and enjoyment,' while the opposite – pain – is usually associated with something highly unpleasant and suffering. If you haven't already guessed, this fifth and final core belief is about our relationships.

'Love Equals Pain' is the negative form in which I first learned of this core belief and could immediately relate to the concept. The opposite – pleasure – seemed a bizarre concept to me, as my relationship interactions until that point had been rather fraught to say the least, swinging between the exhilarating highs of feeling 'in love' to the – what seemed inevitable – lows of fear, anxiety, hurt, pain, suffering, rejection and struggle.

Old Core Belief 5: Love Equals Pain

While some of us seem blessed with happy, loving relationships, for others they are a treacherous battleground! Loving relationships are not exclusive to intimate partners, of course, they can exist between family members, friends, work colleagues and even passing strangers, for example, lovingly helping out in a moment of need. They may be a simple gesture of kindness or just having a laugh together.

When we refer to 'love' here, it doesn't necessarily mean we are 'in love', but more the sense of connection we may have to another or others.

For those of us with a 'love equals pain' belief, our relationships and connections to others can seem programmed for pain and difficulty, whether created externally by others or by ourselves, sabotaging something good. The biggest blueprint for our relationships will come from our early upbringing. How our parents or other authority figures were with each other and how they were with us will programme us to feel and believe that this is 'the way it is'; and we will, as we know, consciously and subconsciously seek out people and situations to repeat the patterns.

For myself, my earliest powerful relationship experience was probably the adoption separation, whereby my nineteen-year-old biological mother nursed me for ten days after my birth and then had to hand me over to the nursing staff and didn't see me for another thirty-five years or so. Knowing the full story now, I completely understand and feel a great deal of empathy for her because she was very much forced into the decision.

But as a ten-day-old baby lying in an adoption clinic in 1965, I can only imagine that I and the other children there with me were totally freaking out, feeling abandoned, rejected, isolated from our mothers. 'Unwanted', 'unloved' and 'disconnected' are all words we can retrospectively attach to very non-verbal feelings from our past, but these experiences then set us up for life. We become unknowingly hypnotized and programmed to find ways to feel the same. *How do we know what 'the one' for us feels like? It is the one who doesn't want us!*

So we end up pursuing relationships with people who do not want us, while rejecting or sabotaging those that do, which makes loving relationships very difficult or challenging at times. Meanwhile, the false idea that love equals pain continues.

Something I find bizarre is what happened when I discovered that my birth mother was searching for me. I always knew I was adopted, it was never an issue, and as far as I was concerned my 'adopted' family *was* my family, parents, sister, grandparents and all. I never doubted it and actually grew up in a very loving environment – there was stress and tension at times, but I always felt loved. And yet, when, aged thirty-five, I read a letter given to me by social services that was from my birth mother, a voice from deep inside spoke so loudly in my mind . . . 'Somebody loves me!' It made no sense at all because I had always been surrounded by very loving family and friends, but somewhere deep inside – probably from just ten days old or so – another part of me clearly had a different viewpoint, and I mention this to highlight how deep or subconsciously some of these ideas can run.

Adoptees are not the only ones who go through this, of course. Children of parents who separate can absorb the pain of the parents' struggles and separations and then subconsciously seek out or expect the same to happen in their own lives, recreating the pattern. In fact, any way in which we can feel pain or hurt in a relationship at a time when we are impressionable and unable to rationalize it, it is possible it will set up a pattern and we will play out the 'love equals pain' idea in our life. Here are some of the common ones that people have told me about when seeking my help:

- Unloving, inattentive mothers
- Absent or unsupportive fathers
- Siblings getting or demanding all the attention
- Alcoholic or drug-addicted family environments
- Violent or aggressive situations
- Erratic behaviours caused by mental health issues
- Parent–child role reversal
- Bullying by siblings, teachers or classmates
- Betrayal, breach of trust and sexual abuse trauma
- Sent away to boarding schools or institutions

All these and more can teach us that love and relationships involve pain, hurt, struggle, loss and betrayal, which we then continue into later life.

So many times, people who have been through trauma and abuse as a child have told me that hurt and pain and suffering is *all they know* in relationships, and it is not until we can access the beliefs, along with any suppressed or repressed emotions, and dehypnotize them from that way of thinking and feeling subconsciously that they can begin to experience something else, something more loving.

Others have told me that, if they do finally find themselves with a loving partner, it triggers angst and discomfort; they display irrational behaviours and mood swings, bringing the pain and hurt into the relationship themselves, subconsciously encouraging the loving partner to treat them in the painful, unloving way they have been expecting. (I have been there and done that one myself with distinction!)

So many times, people have said to me, 'I've finally found someone who loves me and who I want to be with but I'm scared I'll send them away.'

Or worse still, it has already happened and they are left on their own again, having destroyed what could have been a perfectly loving union.

'Love equals pain' causes us to feel heartache, sadness, loss, loneliness, emptiness, hurt, anxiety, guilt and more, and the *fear* of being hurt in this way is often what causes us to display *what seems like* irrational behaviour – but it makes perfect sense when we understand it is just the threat response attempting to protect ourselves or create what feels familiar.

Are we at the mercy of our past? No! Can we break the cycles? Yes, absolutely! As we peel back the layers of fear and limitation, and allow more of the Real You to come through, the more happiness, satisfaction, enjoyment and pleasure you will experience in your relationships.

New Core Belief 5: Love Equals Pleasure

The Real You Knows that Love Equals Pleasure

The Real You – the one without all the fears, limiting ideas and negative programming from life – intrinsically knows that love equals pleasure. The more that Real You comes to the surface, the more you can experience pleasure – a feeling of happiness, satisfaction and enjoyment – in your relationships.

This is not always easy because our relationships can, of course, trigger some of the biggest hurts and pains, but if we can also see them as presenting us with the greatest opportunities to evolve, we can use difficult situations to our advantage. The 'pain' we feel will lead us to our beliefs and if we can face whatever we find there, and deal with it, even the biggest hurt can be a catalyst for change. I'm not saying we should seek that out – but if it happens, we should use it.

And by the way, although there will be times when a change is needed, we don't necessarily always have to leave our current relationship, if we are in one, in order to get what we feel is currently lacking.

Often, when we evolve to a new way of thinking, feeling and behaving, we then begin to bring out different behaviours and attitudes in those around us and with whom we come into contact. Other times, though, as we evolve ourselves, we will feel a natural inclination to move on in some way – whether it be new job, new friends, new partner or whatever.

However it happens, when we begin to carry within us more focus on the idea of love and relationships being about pleasure, our circumstances eventually begin to reflect that.

But as with all issues in our life, first we need to become aware of what is happening so that we can interrupt the old subconscious programming and then begin to introduce new, more satisfactory ideals.

Exercise 14: Awareness of Pain or Pleasure in Relationships

Duration: 10–20 minutes
Journal Required: Yes
Buddy Required: Optional

Background

'Love hurts' is the saying, but it doesn't need to be that way. If we live by the mantra 'love equals pain', we will find ways to experience it that way; when 'love equals pleasure' becomes our mantra, an ancient pain can melt away and we can find people coming into our life to reflect this more positive idea back to us.

To begin with, we need to become aware though.

Instructions

Part 1

1. As we have done before, go back in your journal to our very first 'Awareness of Meaning' exercise, Part 3.
2. Referring to the positive, negative, neutral or mixed responses to the people who came to mind, feel around for any way in which this idea of 'love equals pain' or 'love equals pleasure' is playing out.
3. Pay attention to the *words* you use when you think of each person and write them down in your journal next to their names. For example:

   - J = Kind, loving, supportive
   - L = Annoying, angry, can't be trusted

- G = Cold, distant, like a stone wall
- C = Flaky, weak, useless

Part 2

1. Expand this idea further. On a page in your journal make a list of the major areas of your life where you come into contact with people: Home, Work, Social, Extended Family, Other.
2. For each area, close your eyes for a few moments and feel around inside for any areas where 'love equals pain' is playing itself out, by acknowledging any areas where there is struggle, challenge, difficulty or lack of loving feelings. Feel around also for the opposite, where 'love equals pleasure' and the relationships and connections feel good. For each of these major areas of life, make a note as to whether 'pain' or 'pleasure' seems to be most relevant.
3. Let your mind link and connect to times, scenes and situations you are currently experiencing or have done in the past. You do not have to think of every person – the meaningful ones, relevant to this exercise, will come to mind quite naturally.
4. For each one, make a note of the name in your journal, along with any specific words you associate with each of these relationships. For example:

   - When [name] behaves like [describe behaviour] I feel [describe the feeling].

5. Again, be honest with what you feel inside and the words that come to mind, even if they surprise or shock you.
6. When finished, look out for any repeating words or phrases and circle them to highlight them, both positive and/or negative.

This will help make you more aware of any beliefs operating – consciously or subconsciously – which is important if there are any negative patterns we wish to break.

Part 3

Finally, write out some summary statements of any patterns you notice in your answers from Part 2 and ask yourself a question: 'For [this feeling] to occur with several different people, I may be carrying a belief, or habitually giving meaning to what I experience, to make me feel that way. I wonder what that belief or meaning is?'

Make a note of anything that seems to come to mind but do not sit wracking your brain to think of something. Let it happen naturally or walk away and come back to it later.

And remember – this is not just about negatives. If you find yourself struggling to identify painful relationship patterns, it may be that you actually have very positive ones and so don't even need to question them.

Part 4

If, as you do these exercises, you become aware of any situations or relationships you seem to be *avoiding*, see if you can identify the fear that is driving this avoidance. For example:

- I don't want another relationship because they are just too much hurt and always end in pain. [That is a belief, an opinion, based on experience.]
- I don't [describe what you avoid] because I am afraid of [describe the feeling].

This may seem a bit negative at first, but remember, identifying fears and limitations at the right level is the key to real and lasting change. We will refer back to these answers later and tell you what to do to begin experiencing things differently. For now, we are still sliding down that first side of the U-Flow, digging the ground, preparing the soil and bringing a few weeds to the surface in the process, before we can begin planting out what we want instead and heading back up the other side.

Exercise 15: Increasing Your Sense of 'Love Equals Pleasure'

Duration: 5–10 minutes
Journal Required: Possibly
Buddy Required: Optional

Background

When life has taught us that love equals pain, we will find ways to bring that into our relationships; when we can remind ourselves that love is really about pleasure, we can find greater happiness, satisfaction and enjoyment.

Instructions

As with previous similar exercises, you can do the following exercise by reading and remembering it; by making a recording using a voice note on your phone; by having an E.S.C.A.P.E. Buddy read it to you; or do the relaxation and focus bit first of all, then open your eyes and read the ideas to yourself, closing your eyes afterwards to let them sink in.

1. Find somewhere quiet, take a few long, slow breaths, as before, relaxing your shoulders on the exhale.
2. Make the out-breath longer than the in-breath, so that it feels like a very gentle sigh of relief, as in earlier exercises.
3. Close your eyes as you breathe out and go within, allowing the muscles of your body to relax as you do.
4. Maintain the breathing for several more of these sigh-of-relief-type breaths.

5. As you do, pay attention to any thoughts that come up for you, but as you breathe out, imagine blowing them away and refocusing your attention on your breath.
6. Tell your body to *relax*.
7. After a few more normal breaths, let your mind focus deeper within yourself and feel around for a place deep within, away from the normal world, beyond the thoughts and fears and limitations of your life. Feel around inside for somewhere safe, with a feeling of deep, deep peace, or the idea of it at the very least.
8. Take as long as you need to do this. It will get quicker and easier each time you do.
9. Once you feel calmer or have a sense of this deep peace within you, say to yourself three times:

> *The Real Me does not seek out painful relationships, the Real Me seeks loving relationships, invites loving people into my life and brings out loving qualities in others.*
> *The Real Me equates love and relationships with pleasure.*
> *The Real Me is love.*

You can repeat this as many times as you wish, or rephrase to make it more specific to your own situation, but as before, it is not about the words – it is about the *feeling* they create and what they are helping you to reach for.

Does this mean you will wake up tomorrow feeling like you're in a yogurt and fresh fruit commercial, with gleaming white kitchen, rainbow-coloured food, white smiling teeth and dazzling white clothing with sunlight pouring through the window? Who knows! But what will happen is you will begin to break the old patterns of negative expectations, plant the seed of doubt with regards to the old way of thinking and pave the way for something new. New may be new people or new may be a new connection to the current people, or both.

Here is a simpler version you can use through the day. Any time you are feeling 'pain' associated with any kind of relationship, imagine a big red 'STOP' sign, take a deep breath and, as you breathe out, say to yourself:

The Real Me seeks loving relationships, invites loving people into my life and brings out loving qualities in others.

Resistance

If you find this exercise difficult or experience resistance, again that is OK, but see if you can identify the resistance. Ask yourself, 'What am I afraid of here about accepting loving relationships for myself?'

In your journal, be sure to make a note of any answer in the following format: 'I am afraid of accepting that the Real Me can have happy, loving, pleasurable, satisfying and enjoyable relationships now because . . .'

And don't be surprised if the answer is actually connected to one of the other core beliefs. For example, some of us are afraid to think about loving relationships because we do not feel good enough for that – or they do not make us feel safe – or we may feel out of control or fear being not accepted and rejected instead.

As we explore further, you will discover how all these beliefs are interconnected, but for now, let's just take a look at the final stage of the E.S.C.A.P.E. Method, which describes what we can experience as a result of advancements in any of the first five key areas of 'Enoughness', Safeness, Control, Acceptance and Pleasure.

E for EN-LIGHTENMENT

In Buddhism, enlightenment is often referred to as 'the end of suffering', and whenever I am working with someone one-to-one, I often check in to see how they are feeling as we progress through the session to find out how much of their 'suffering' we have been able to ease. One of the simplest ways to get an honest and direct answer is to ask them to notice how their body feels because their body will be responding to both their conscious and subconscious thoughts. Maybe the body even is the sub-conscious mind because it can certainly seem that way at times.

Whenever I have been able to help someone ease one of their old core beliefs, in whichever area of life they are seeking change, and enable them to feel more of their real, positive self, there is something I've noticed about the way they describe how their body feels afterwards: **'It feels lighter and free. *I* feel lighter and free, like a burden has been lifted.'**

It happened so often, I actually began to use this as a measure as to how well the session had gone. If they felt lighter and free – en-lightened – we had achieved a successful outcome. If not, there was still some work to do.

Feeling en-lightened is the result I am looking for when I take people through the E.S.C.A.P.E. Method and it is one of the aims of my writing this book. At the very least to help you make progress or become more aware; at best to feel a deep sense of this yourself.

If you think back to the U-Flow diagram, one of the challenges is to fig-ure out at what level we actually need to operate in order to bring about the change we desire, and I placed core beliefs at the bottom, as the foundation. However, as we start to apply these into more specific areas of your life, you will see that they are playing out at all levels – from the surface-level symptoms to beliefs to any traumatic memories you hold, and deeper still.

If you think back over the exercises we have been doing around 'Enoughness', Safeness, Control, Acceptance and Pleasure, these are the ideas I am looking for when I first begin chatting with someone in a one-to-one client session.

Sometimes a simple shift in perspective will be enough to facilitate the change and help the client feel lighter, freer and unburdened; sometimes we will have to take that person on a journey through emotionally charged memories and beliefs. If there has been a lot of trauma or upset, we may have to do this a number of times, clearing different layers each time.

We may start out with clearing the past and then gradually transition to more solution-focused approaches as the major traumas get eased, and we can merely fine-tune things on the surface. Or, conversely, as life gets better and better, we may need to get progressively deeper to reach where we need to – it all depends on the individual.

As you work through these exercises yourself, and the ones that follow, you may find you have similar experiences.

We never actually *need* to dig into the past, remember, because really it is only the *effect* of the past we are interested in, but releasing suppressed or repressed emotion in this way can be a very fast way to bring about deep and lasting transformations, creating that lightness we are looking for.

Whichever way we go through this process, any time we identify and release a limiting idea, we are moving away from the conditioning and limitations in our life, dehypnotizing ourselves from life's programming and becoming more of that person we were born to be. The Real You, who has been patiently waiting to be discovered, or rediscovered, can finally 'E.S.C.A.P.E.' and be free.

Sometimes I describe it as like taking off a pair of spectacles that have been putting a filter on life for you; when removed, they suddenly allow you a whole new level of experience that was always there but was filtered out, and didn't seem available until now. Or, conversely, like being given a new pair that allow you to see properly for the first time in a long time!

The Real You is En-Lightened

Feeling 'en-lightened' is not about achieving a deep mystical state in order to escape life – it is about letting go of fears, limitations, false beliefs, illusions, doubts and conditioned responses so that we can fully *embrace* life.

The surface-level you, who has been reacting and adapting because of various levels of threat response and conditioning, is the one who experiences moments of pleasure and happiness amidst a stream of everyday problems, varying in intensity depending on your individual circumstances.

The Real You is en-lightened – again, not by achieving some magical state, but already, naturally, intrinsically, inherently so. To experience it, we just need to clear away the ideas that have been making us feel the opposite. As a result of a step-by-step process of challenging and changing our core beliefs, facing our fears, feeling what we really feel and focusing on who we really are underneath, everything begins to change. We feel different, we feel lighter, we feel freer, and that emanates into all areas of our life, impacting how we think, feel and behave, the choices we make and the outcomes we experience as a result.

Do we always have to go through this E.S.C.A.P.E. Method in order to feel this? Not at all. I am merely giving you a structure to follow for something that is actually very fluid and open to spontaneity and endless possibilities. But a shift in one or more of the core beliefs will always precede a feeling of en-lightenment, however it comes about.

Although sometimes we can take dramatic leaps, when using self-help it is usually a more gentle unfolding, an easing, a letting go, so that something which previously troubled us can now become harmless or meaningless, a relic even, like shedding an old heavy overcoat that we no longer need on a hot, sunny day.

I have spent a lot of my life trying to run away from what *is* in an attempt to find that something *more*, out there. There were definitely times when change was needed, but what it has taken me so long to realize is that the Real Me, the one I was desperately trying to find 'out there', was in the mirror staring back at me all along, and in the eyes of every person I have ever met. I only had to look in the right way.

The Real You, en-lightened, happy, free, is there in the mirror looking back at you as well, and in the eyes of every person you meet. You, too, only have to look in the right way.

There is one more exercise we need do on this to further cement the ideas thus far and then we can begin to move on to how to relate these, at times, rather lofty concepts to details and specifics of your everyday life.

Exercise 16: Increasing Your Sense of En-lightenment

Duration: 5–10 minutes
Journal Required: Possibly
Buddy Required: Optional

Background

When we transform any of our core beliefs from the negative to the positive version and apply that to the area of life that has been troubling us, our previous suffering will begin to ease and we will feel lighter and freer.

Instructions

Follow the instructions, as with previous exercises, in the best way that you've found works for you.

1. Find somewhere quiet, take a few long, slow breaths, as before, relaxing your shoulders on the exhale.
2. Make the out-breath longer than the in-breath, so that it feels like a very gentle sigh of relief, as in earlier exercises.
3. Close your eyes as you breathe out and go within, allowing the muscles of your body to relax as you do.
4. Maintain the breathing for several more of these sigh-of-relief-type breaths.
5. As you do, pay attention to any thoughts that come up for you, but as you breathe out, imagine blowing them away and refocusing your attention on your breath.
6. Tell your body to *relax*.

7. After a few more normal breaths, let your mind focus deeper within yourself and feel around for a place deep within, away from the normal world, beyond the thoughts and fears and limitations of your life. Feel around inside for somewhere safe, with a feeling of deep, deep peace, or the idea of it at the very least.

8. Take as long as you need to do this. It will get quicker and easier each time you do.

9. Once you feel calmer or have a sense of this idea of deep peace within you, think about the five core beliefs and imagine how different life could feel for you if these statements were now true, in the positive versions.

The Positive Versions

*Even though I may have found it difficult
to accept or believe until now . . .*

The Real Me is enough – worthy, valid – exactly as I am, right
here, right now, unquestionably, even before I have done those things
I think I need to do to earn the right or prove I am enough.*

*The Real Me is safe and is able to project that outwards, so that
the world is a safe place for me to live, work and operate.
The Real Me feels safe, even before I have done
those things I think I need to do to be safe.*

*The Real Me is strong, powerful and in control, able to
adapt and evolve to the twists and turns of life.
The Real Me can feel comfortably in control, even without
needing to be overcontrolling of myself or others or life.*

* If you feel more comfortable changing 'I' and 'Me' to 'You' when repeating these statements to yourself, at least at first, it's fine to do so.

> *I can accept the Real Me and as a result the Real Me feels*
> *accepted, fits in, belongs, has a place, a purpose,*
> *is connected, exactly as I am.*
> *I can welcome the Real Me with open arms, not in spite of who*
> *I really am but because of who I really am [think about that!],*
> *without needing to change anything, and as a result feel*
> *accepted by life, in the same way.*
>
> *The Real Me knows love as pleasure and seeks relationships*
> *and connections which reflect that. The Real Me finds happiness,*
> *satisfaction and enjoyment in relationships, even*
> *without having to sacrifice who I am.*
>
> *Free of the heaviness of fear and limitation*
> *And free of the fear of not being enough.*
> *Free of the fear of attack from an unsafe world 'out there'*
> *And free of the fear of losing control.*
> *Free of the fear of judgement and exclusion*
> *And free of the idea that love equals pain.*
> *The Real Me is En-lightened*
> *And Free, able to fully love and embrace life*
> *And all it offers.*

You can repeat these statements as many times as you wish, but as we have said before, it is not about the words – it is about the *feeling* they create, and what they are helping you to reach for.

Here is a simpler version you can use through the day, any time you are feeling stress or tension. Imagine a big red 'STOP' sign, take a deep breath and, as you breathe out, say to yourself:

The Real Me does not need to feel this. The Real Me can feel light and free, whenever I am ready to allow it.

When we 'allow it', as the club owner, we are effectively changing the door policy so that ideas our critical faculty would previously have rejected can now be allowed in.

Resistance

If you feel any resistance, that is OK. Sometimes it can take a lot of repetition and focus to overwrite a lifetime of programming and conditioning. But we do not want to just keep trying to run up a down escalator, of course. In the exercises that follow, we will seek to dissolve resistance further, and one thing that can cause us to feel resistance to allowing change, even when we know something is not right and not good for us, is a loss of identity. We will look at this in the next chapter.

Who Are You? What is Your True Identity?

If you refer back to the U-Flow diagram again (p. 112), you will see that all of those various elements, from core beliefs through life experiences to individual beliefs and the thoughts, feelings, emotions and behaviours that arise from them, create an overall identity.

Identity is really important when we are seeking to bring about change because our behaviour will nearly always follow our identity, and if we try to change something that goes against an old identity, this too can create resistance and prevent us completing the U-Flow and coming back up the other side.

But what do we really mean by identity?

In one definition our identity is the way in which the world can identify us – our name is a part of our identity, for example, and there are many people who change their name when changing how they want to be seen by the world. This may be a permanent change when going through a major transition in life or a temporary one as we take on different roles each day, meandering our way through our home, family, social and working life.

As I mentioned earlier, back in the early 1990s I was a guitarist and another band I played for was theatrical punk-rock outfit Jonah and The Wail. On stage, with bleached blond hair, leather jacket and low-slung guitar, surrounded by flashing lights, smoke and noise, I was introduced as 'The Feedback Monster'! Seems comical now, but it fit the situation well and my behaviour on stage followed that identity – strutting, arrogant, aggressive, provocative.

But if I used that name – or identity – outside of that environment – at the dentist, for example – for me it would have felt ridiculous: 'Good morning, Mr Monster, what can we do for you today?' 'Er, please, just call me Andrew.'

Many of us will take on an External Identity in order to help us cope or deal with situations. We may identify with a certain type of music or culture and dress to fit in; we may dress to impress; or to shock; or to be invisible. In fact, we may take on any number of External Identities, depending on how our core beliefs are playing out.

All these external coping identities are OK, of course, but they tend to be temporary and perishable. For me, the highs of being on stage and performing were often followed by terrible lows, with feelings of shame, self-loathing and wanting to hide away. I believe this is because there was a conflict of identities created by a sense of my lack of worth; outwardly I was acting out one thing (fight), but inwardly I was feeling something else (flight), and would swing between the two extremes, each one trying to compensate for the other.

Over the years, as I have resolved the underlying issues and allowed my self-worth and self-esteem to increase, I have gradually let go of both previous false identities, so that now when I need to perform – whether giving a speech, teaching in front of a group of students or occasionally performing on a stage, as I still enjoy doing – in each of the situations, both on and off the stage, I am being myself – the same, more authentic, natural self. My inner and outer are much more aligned, just different expressions of the Real Me.

Any time we take on a false identity in order to compensate for something, there is a risk of being found out. Nowadays we often hear of people suffering from Imposter Syndrome, which typically occurs when people are given a promotion or offered a job they feel underqualified or inexperienced to perform, and worry that at some point they will be found out. This triggers the threat response so the work or situation becomes stressful rather than an enjoyable experience.

Very often, once again, this will be owing to limiting beliefs picked up from childhood or life experiences, causing us to doubt our worth or value; we are afraid of people seeing what we think is the 'real' us – one that is 'not enough' for the role. We think, 'Inwardly I feel scared, anxious, not good enough, on the verge of being exposed, ashamed and ridiculed, but if I look the part, say the right things and get the job done . . . I might just get away with it!'

We might get away with it . . . for a while. But those pesky beliefs have a habit of finding their way to the surface and making themselves known. Eventually, inevitably, a crack will appear and our worst nightmare will seem to be about to come true.

But if we are honest with ourselves – really honest – then those moments can actually be major turning points. Interestingly, when we can be brave enough to let our External Identity fall away and allow something of the natural, real, authentic self to shine through, something magical usually happens. Instead of the ridicule, shame and rejection we may have been expecting, we actually get love, acceptance, endearment . . . and freedom.

When I first moved to my Harley Street office, in London, I remember thinking, 'I suppose I had better wear a suit now and dress a bit smarter' – Harley Street being one of the UK and world's most exclusive medical addresses.

But then I thought, 'Who am I wearing a suit for? Who am I trying to impress?' So instead, I decided to wear jeans and a sweatshirt to work, to force myself to be me, rather than something I was trying to be.

On the train on the way to the clinic that first day I remember glancing down, seeing my jeans, and for a split-second panicked – 'Huh, I forgot to get dressed properly!' And then I remembered. At first, I felt nervous, anxious, vulnerable, open, exposed. I imagined all sorts of scenarios where I opened the door to clients and they made disparaging remarks. But, instead, something very different happened.

As I simply decided to be myself, I noticed that the clients in suits would start to dress down as they came in, taking their tie off, sliding their jacket over their shoulder, adapting to me and my dress code. Others would breathe a sigh of relief, seeing a relatively normal-looking person instead of their expectation of a serious 'professional', and their guard would lower.

And for me it felt so much easier going to work – less like work – just going out for the day to chat to some people and see if I could help them. The less I had to *be* something, the more I could be me.

But to do this I also had to face my old Inner Identity – and this is where the major challenge often arises. When we adopt a certain External Identity we are usually doing so to protect or compensate for an inner one we are seeking to hide. When we no longer fear our Inner Identity being exposed, we no longer need the external one to protect it.

My own Inner Identity at the time had been saying, 'Being me is not quite enough – so I had better do something external [i.e. wear a smart suit] to make up for that.' When I challenged that idea and took some positive action to reinforce the new idea, I went through some temporary emotional discomfort as I faced the fear, but then slowly my beliefs updated and dressing more casually became normal. My actions helped develop a new belief, but my risking my acceptance of myself as I am gave me the courage and commitment to do it.

Even though certain beliefs and identities may be causing us problems, we often have an emotional investment in sustaining them – and will even go to great lengths to defend them! Think of how vigorously people stand up for their religious or political identity, which is no more than a collection of strongly held ideas, beliefs or opinions.

Remember, we will have internal references – memories and life experiences – to 'prove' why our beliefs and identity are valid and need to be maintained. Any attempt at challenging the identity head on, without being aware of the beliefs supporting it, risks triggering the threat response, which will create resistance to change.

There will be an *identity* associated with *the area we wish to change*. And there may be resistance to letting go of that identity, which we will need to take care of.

So back to the original question: Who are you? What is your true identity? Our honest answer to this is really key to our ability to escape the limitations of our lives. If we cannot even admit to ourselves who or what we think we are, we will never be able to change and will always be left seeking something external to protect or compensate for how we feel on the inside.

When we can face up to who – or what – we think we are, and find the courage to reveal and believe in a new identity, a form of Identity Switch can occur, whereby we can often experience rapid change.

CASE STUDY: *Ten Days in Ten Seconds*

As an example of how an Identity Switch can help us make quite dramatic changes, this case study relates to one of my practitioner training attendees who casually mentioned he wanted to give up smoking because he felt like a liar, running a voluntary group to help people with addictions in the evening but still 'addicted' to smoking himself.

'You're right!' I said, looking him straight in the eyes, latching on to his Identity Statement. 'You are a liar.'

One of the other attendees looked a bit shocked, asking, 'Are we allowed to say that?'

I don't usually go around calling people liars but since he had used that phrase to define himself in that way – 'I am a liar' – and I could see where he was coming from, rather than reassure him, I thought I would just call him out on it and see if we could flip it round.

He seemed to appreciate the honesty, and when I asked him when he was going to quit, he started talking but avoided answering. When he had finished, I asked him again, 'When are you going to quit?'

Again, he started talking, this time about the system he had used before to stop smoking, which involved 'ten days of misery or struggle' and writing things down. I just asked him again, 'If it could happen very easily, without all that struggle and suffering, when would be a good time to quit?'

'Well, now,' he said, which was the answer I was looking for. But although I could see he was sincere, I still needed a hook, a big enough why, to make it easier for him to stay committed.

'Instead of being a *liar*,' I said, emphasizing the word 'liar', which was part of his old smoker identity, 'what would you rather be instead?'

'An inspirer!' he said after a few moments' consideration, and now I had the fuel we needed for the Identity Switch.

'OK, so when are you ready to become an inspirer?' I asked, shifting the focus away from the old smoking habit, wanting it to be something undesirable from the past that he could let go of.

'Now,' he answered emphatically, and much more quickly.

I was about to say to him, 'Look, what you achieved in ten days before need only take ten minutes now. And what you can achieve in ten minutes need only take ten seconds, if you are ready and willing.' But I never got the chance because he was already reaching into his pocket and handing me his cigarettes.

'Are you sure?' I checked, wanting to make sure the decision came from him, not me.

'Absolutely,' he replied. 'Keep them!'

Later that evening I texted him a short message, reminding him that the only thing he needed was a deep breath in and out of his mouth (thus simulating the action of smoking, to help reduce the idea of there being something missing for a while), and that he was an inspirer.

What had taken ten days of suffering previously had taken less than ten seconds once he felt able to switch identity and had a good enough reason to do so. As an inspirer, his new behaviours could now follow that new identity.

Catching up with him several months later, he explained how he had remained smoke-free for a month or so after the exchange, but then a stressful incident had triggered him starting again. However, he now felt closer to letting go once more and realized it could be a simple and natural process when he was fully ready.

Breaking habits can be a long and arduous process if we are fighting against ourselves – but if we have the right motivation and the right belief, old habits can fall away in an instant, especially if we are able to switch identity: 'I was this but now I am this – so now, I do this!'

One of the aims of the E.S.C.A.P.E. Method is to take you down one side of the U-Flow and peel away old layers of beliefs and identity so that you can come up the other side transformed, lighter and freer, with a new identity, closer to the Real You, that is in alignment with your desired outcomes.

Exercise 17: Awareness of Your Identities

Duration: 15–20 minutes
Journal Required: Yes
Buddy Required: Optional

Background

As we switch roles in life we often take on different identities. All of these are designed to serve or protect us in some way, but if they are there to 'protect' the Real You, rather than be an expression of the Real You, then we are likely to experience fear, anxiety and stress at times. Becoming aware of this is the first step to helping us break free of any identities that no longer serve us.

Instructions

1. On a new page in your journal, headed 'Awareness of Identities', make a note of the various External Identities you portray to others as you take on various roles throughout your daily life. What is your identity at home? With family? At work? With friends? With colleagues? Playing or watching sports? Is part of your identity linked to religious or spiritual affiliations or your nationality? For example:

   - At home I am [the 'clever one'] . . .
   - At work I am [the boss] . . .
   - With my spouse I am [the gofer!] . . .
   - With my friends I am [the funny one] . . .
   - At college I am [the student] . . .

2. For each one, make a note of any way in which you have connected these roles or identities to any of your core beliefs, for example:

   - Which ones give you a sense of self-worth and value?
   - Which ones help you feel safe and secure?
   - Which ones help you feel strong, powerful and in control?
   - Which ones help you feel a part of something, loved, accepted, belonging?
   - Which ones give you pleasure?

3. Feel around inside for what you have been thinking of as the 'real you' until now, which may be an aspect of yourself you have been keeping hidden.

4. Think about all the roles and identities you portray from Step 1 and think about any fears you have of anyone in those circumstances finding out about what you have been thinking of as the 'real you' until now.

5. Make a note in your journal of any way you have had to hide a part of yourself to fulfil that role; or have had to step up in some way and try to be something you feel you are not; or would feel uncomfortable if others could see.

6. Feel around for any areas where you may have been taking on an External Identity in order to hide from or compensate for an Inner Identity, and write it out, long-form, like this:

   • I have been taking on [this External Identity] because inwardly I feel [. . .] and have been afraid that [. . .].

   NOTE: Do not judge yourself – just become aware. Remember, the aim is simply to make the invisible visible.

7. For any areas mentioned in Step 6, write out and complete the following statement:

   • If I could be the Real Me (i.e. the one who is free of fear and limitations) then instead of [. . .] I could/would [. . .].

Our Behaviour Follows Our Identity

One day, in the middle of a Question and Answer session at one of my early practitioner classes, somebody asked me, 'Why do you snap your fingers to bring someone back after a session?'

To which I replied, 'Because I am a hypnotist,' and everybody laughed. But it was true, at that time.

I used to do that little snapping fingers thing to encourage people to open their eyes at the end of a session not because I particularly needed to, it was just what people like me did in situations like that, and that was who I thought I was. It was a behaviour that went with my identity at the time.

And the same is true for all of us in many areas of life. Our beliefs have created identities, which have become a part of who we are, and our behaviours then follow: 'This is who I am – so this is what I do.'

Our behaviours will always follow our identity – not necessarily the other way round – which can add a surprising twist to self-analysis of our behaviours.

- Am I a smoker because I smoke?
- Or do I smoke because I believe I am a smoker?

- Am I overweight because I overeat?
- Or do I overeat because I believe I am overweight?

- Am I dissatisfied in my relationship because there is no love and care?
- Or is there no love and care because I identify myself as someone for whom relationships are dissatisfying in that way?

Some of this may seem backwards at first but as we unravel what is really happening and reveal the programming behind it, very often we see that it is our *self-definition* that creates the behaviours and experiences rather than our behaviours and experiences creating our self-definition.

But this leaves us with another potential problem to face or resolve, as I mentioned briefly earlier. What if our new desired behaviour or way of being contradicts a long-held belief about ourselves and our core identity – the way we see or define ourselves as a person? This will leave us in conflict, trying to run up that down escalator again, because it is very difficult to sustain any change within ourselves if we maintain an old identity that contradicts or conflicts with the new, more desired way of being.

- If I am a smoker, I must smoke, so how can I stop smoking?
- If I am lazy, I don't do exercise, so how can I get fit and lose the weight I want to?
- If I am the party animal, I must get really drunk, so how can I get sober and sort my life out?
- If I am a loner, I stay away from others, so how can I form the loving relationship I secretly yearn for?
- If I am [identity label], I [behave in a certain way], so how can I [achieve the result I want] if I now need to think, feel or do something that contradicts that?

But what if we could be willing to change our identity in some way? To change who we think we are or how we label ourselves? What could happen then, do you think? A lasting change in behaviour or being will often require a simultaneous shift in identity and it is an acceptance of the shift in identity that will actually allow the change to be lasting.

Interestingly, adopting a new identity is often a very rapid way to liberate ourselves from old ways of thinking, feeling and behaving, and allow new, more desirable thoughts, feelings and behaviours to come to the surface instead – provided there is no deeper conflict, of course.

At first this may seem like a great shortcut. Why bother with all that other stuff about core beliefs and memories and emotions, etc., if we can just switch identity?

The answer is in the last line of the previous paragraph: 'provided there is no deeper conflict'.

We cannot just give ourselves a new identity and expect it to last if we secretly harbour contradictory thoughts, feelings, emotions and beliefs because they will eventually rise to the surface and, if unchallenged, cause the new identity to break down.

However, if we can create a new identity and then align all our thoughts, feelings, beliefs and behaviours to that, including challenging and resolving any resistance that comes up, our new identity can endure.

When dealing with a little habit like smoking or nail-biting, for example, the habitual behaviour itself is of little relevance to me in the discussion. My focus is on understanding the person's beliefs around it and helping them create a new identity as a non-smoker or someone who takes care of their nails or whatever the desired change may be.

If I am a smoker, I must smoke, and any attempt not to will create conflict and be like asking me to go against my identity, which requires effort and 'willpower' – this is the real reason why so many people find it difficult to stop smoking.

If, however, I am a non-smoker, things are very different. Non-smokers, by definition, do not smoke and therefore not smoking is easy as long as I adopt the new identity. People say, 'Yes, but what about the addiction?' to which I reply, there is no addiction if the person can sufficiently adopt the new identity – because the addiction belonged to the old identity, along with any fears, anxieties and limiting beliefs that went with it.

When we can do this – when we can adopt the new identity that is more fitting of the changes we desire – our subconscious mind helps us to make new choices and generates new behaviours to reflect this, which then make it easier or more likely to create the right conditions for what we prefer.

So a large part of the dehypnotizing process we need to go through in order to solve our problems is dissolving of an old identity and replacing it with a new one. Or allowing a new one to naturally form as the old one falls away. But, again, it cannot be just an intellectual exercise. To be sustained, the change has to occur at all levels, from the surface-level symptoms right the way down to the core beliefs.

We formed our old beliefs and old identity over time through a process of natural hypnosis and conditioning from life, and we can use the very same natural phenomenon to reverse the process. By simply allowing our minds to relax, focus and go inward, into a state of natural hypnosis, we can access the thoughts, feelings, memories, beliefs and ideas that have been creating the old identity – not to brainwash, but to un-brainwash and *restore* a better way of thinking, one that has been there all along, just waiting to shine through. We can allow a new, more evolved identity to emerge – the Real You – one befitting of the new version of ourselves we are seeking to become.

As we release the old identity and accept the new, our thoughts, feelings, behaviours, choices and outcomes will change accordingly and we will now be more likely to make the right decisions and take the appropriate actions to create the right conditions to bring about the more desired outcome.

Whether helping people break simple habits, achieve major goals or create deep and lasting transformations in their life, I am nearly always looking for an 'I am' shift in identity to assist the process. 'I was *this* . . . but now I am THIS!' Once we have that, a natural cascade of new ideas and behaviours can follow, as this new identity can begin to play itself out in the details of everyday life. We can say that any statement we make about ourselves that begins with 'I am [this] . . .' is an Identity Statement.

Exercise 18: How to Reveal Your Invisible Identities

Duration: 48 hours
Journal Required: Yes
Buddy Required: No

Background

Earlier on we did an exercise on becoming aware of the identities we may carry within us attached to the typical roles we play in life. Now we will dig a little deeper and explore if we can reveal some of the invisible ones – identities that are operating in plain sight but out of our awareness.

Instructions

Part 1

1. On a new page in your journal, write the heading 'Hidden Identities'.
2. Underneath that write a subheading, 'I Am This . . . So I Do This'.
3. Now divide the page into two columns, labelled as below:

<u>I Am This</u>   <u>So I Do This</u>

4. For the next twenty-four hours, make a note of every time you say or think anything that involves, or is related to, an 'I am' statement that refers to some kind of description about yourself, and write it under the 'I Am This' heading. So you would include 'I am so lazy' but you would not include 'I am going to the shops' unless the action had a direct meaning in relation to an aspect of yourself. Be aware also of any labels around roles, cultural beliefs, political beliefs, religious or spiritual beliefs.
5. Then, in the opposite column, write down what you actually do that makes you say this about yourself: 'I am this . . . so I do this.'

For example:

<u>I Am This</u>	<u>So I Do This</u>
I am so stupid	I must keep making mistakes
I am forgetful	I must keep forgetting things
I'm shy	I must feel nervous talking to people
I am tired	I must run out of energy or concentration
I am late	I must not leave enough time
I am overweight	I must eat more than I need
I am useless	I must seek experiences to prove that

| I am a victim | I must seek experiences in which I can feel victimized |
| I am a [label] | I must seek/behave in accordance with that label |

Keep adding to the list for a full forty-eight hours and do not exclude any thought or observation – if it comes to mind or into your awareness, write it down.

At first it may seem weird or as if we are stating the obvious, but what we are seeking to pick up on are the comments and self-talk 'labels' that you say to yourself – unchallenged – that will go right past your critical faculty and reinforce an existing idea about yourself. Behaviour follows identity, so if at some level we feel and believe ourselves to be these things – stupid, forgetful, tired, shy, late, for example – we will subconsciously act in a way to perpetuate more of the same.

Part 2

Now repeat the exercise but in reverse.

1. Still under the main heading of 'Hidden Identities', write a new subheading, 'I Do This . . . So I Am This'.
2. Now you are going to become very aware of the way you behave and make a note of what you do first . . . and then think about why you are doing it and any way in which you could give yourself a label for that.

For example:

I Do This	So I Am This
I am checking my phone every few minutes	I am an anxious parent
I am checking the lights five times before I go out for the day	I have OCD
I am smoking a cigarette	I am a smoker

I am getting angry with my children	I am impatient
I am running around helping everybody	I am the supportive one
I am eating more than I need when feeling sad or upset	I am a comfort eater
I am getting nervous about speaking in public	I am a nervous public speaker
I [feel/do/experience] this	I am [this]

Part 3

1. Think about the following statement: 'Every time I acquire a label, I acquire a limitation.'
2. Now think about each of the 'I am . . .' Identity Statements from both parts of the exercise and imagine you have been programmed or conditioned by life to think, feel and behave in accordance with those, and that anything outside of them is not allowed or may even trigger the threat response, causing you to conform once again.

   Can you understand why identity – and labels – are so important when seeking to create change? If the transformation we seek means we will need to act outside a current label or Identity Statement in order to avoid conflict, *we must also update the label and statement.*
3. Looking through the 'I am' Identity Statements (labels) from your list, I wonder what different choices, actions and outcomes it might open up for you if you were *free* of them?
4. In your journal, for each Identity Statement, write down: 'Without this old label or identity I could . . .' and pay attention to how you feel as you do.

Are you still tempted to cling to an old identity? If so, why? What does it give you? Which of the core beliefs is it helping to sustain? What would you need to know, feel or believe in order to be able to *finally* let it go now, so that you can evolve, form a NEW identity and move on?

Or are you ready to make an Identity Switch now? Are you ready to allow something new to form, something more in alignment with what you want from the next phase of your life, whatever that is?

In the exercises so far we have been focusing on becoming aware of the impact of our core beliefs and identities in general areas of our life and I hope you can understand why I often dig for these as opposed to just dealing with surface-level symptoms.

Now, while we have been planting the seed for some new ideas here and there, we have largely been making our way down the left-hand side of the U-Flow, which is often very revealing, but definitely the not-so-fun side! But this is only the first half of the E.S.C.A.P.E. Method. What we need to do now is begin to move back up the other side, towards our original destination of improved outcomes.

We need to take the general concepts we have been learning and apply them to more specific, everyday situations so that we can help ease or solve some of our more specific, everyday problems. In so doing, we can move closer to our personal goals and ambitions, whether that be easing an old habit or completely reinventing ourselves with a NEW identity.

Let's begin by getting to grips with what, for me, is one of the absolute basic, but essential, tools for personal change.

Don't Want/Do Want

As I mentioned briefly earlier, when I ask people how I can help them they will usually answer with an 'away' or 'towards' response, telling me either something they want to stop, reduce or get rid of (their 'Don't Want') or something they want to get, be or have more of (their 'Do Want'), and they will have good reasons for wanting these things.

Interestingly, I noticed that whichever side of the Don't Want/Do Want (DW/DW) statement they put forward, they often had great difficulty or resistance to verbalizing the other side. So if they told me about something they 'Don't Want', they often had trouble verbalizing what they 'Do Want'. And if they happily told me what it was they 'Do Want', they were often reluctant or resistant to clarifying what they 'Don't Want'. So I started to pay attention to this and began digging around to see if it had any value hidden within. It did.

Often, when I pushed them to clarify the other side of the statement, we would get an immediate shift in perspective and the problem would be eased in that moment.

If we take the example of people who bite their nails, they would usually tell me that they would like to stop biting their nails – that was their 'Don't Want'. Rarely did they come to me prepared for what they 'Do Want' – which was to leave their nails alone so their nails could heal, repair, restore, grow and become healthy, strong and normal-looking.

Tie this in to an Identity Switch – from 'I am someone who tears and rips at my nails' to 'I am someone who takes care of my nails because they are precious' – and we have a pretty good chance that this person will begin to leave their nails alone so they can grow longer and remain healthy. Connect that to whichever of the core beliefs is most appropriate – Control? 'Enoughness'? Acceptance? – and embed the whole thing by helping the person to relax and focus with their eyes closed, feeling, sensing, picturing and imagining the ideas, and – provided the critical faculty has no objection – we can generally have a super-high success rate, pretty quickly, possibly with a little booster if required. And the same applies for almost any habit.

Other times, however, especially where more emotive issues were concerned, when I asked them to verbalize or express the other side of the DW/DW statement they would become uncomfortable, burst into tears or have an instant release of suppressed or repressed emotions. Such abreactive moments can be extremely cathartic and act as a catalyst for deep and lasting change.

Other times, still, when a client started talking, they would simply pour out a monologue about what they had been through, not actually knowing what they wanted or didn't want! In these cases, I noticed that if we could start with a 'Don't Want', it was usually then easier to find the 'Do Want', so that we could help to create positive ideas around that.

But whichever way round it begins, I always want to know BOTH sides of the equation because that will usually help us get the deepest transformation, with the most lasting result.

So we have a nice, neat and tidy technique that can transform our lives:

1. Find out what we 'Don't Want' – our undesirable surface-level symptoms.
2. Find the exact or near exact *opposite* – what we 'Do Want' instead.
3. Turn that 'Do Want' into some kind of positive mantra that can be reinforced through focus, repetition, visualization and the many techniques available to us.
4. Have a big enough 'Why' to help us overcome any resistance or make it worthwhile exploring deeper if need be.
5. Create a new identity to support the idea, who thinks, feels and behaves differently to before and in alignment with this new idea, which then gets reinforced (conditioned) by Hebbian Learning.

That's it. Simple, right? Sometimes, yes, it really can be that simple.

DON'T WANT	DO WANT
To bite my nails	To take care of my nails
To drink too much	To stay sober
To overdramatize, always imagining the worst	To evaluate what is actually happening and focus on that

These 'Do Wants' can form simple mantras or affirmations that can actually work, especially if you can make them into a form of Identity Statement, whereby the behaviours will follow:

- I am someone who can and does take care of my nails.
- I am someone who stays sober.
- I am someone who evaluates what is actually happening and stays calm and focused.
- I am someone who can and does eat in a way that means I remain slim and healthy.
- I am someone who can and does allow myself satisfying relationships.

To begin with these may seem alien (remember 'Affirmations or Lies?' p. 63) but if there are no contradictory beliefs and we can reinforce these new ideas *without our critical faculty triggering the threat response*, then gently, over time, these new ideas will help to form a new identity, and our behaviours and experiences will then more easily follow to support that.

It can work the other way too: if we focus on these ideas and follow the new behaviours enough, they then become the new normal and we forge a new identity from our behaviour.

How long does it take to build a new habit? Studies seem to change their opinion every few years. To me, it takes as long as it takes to update the beliefs and build the new neural pathways. That may be months, weeks, days, hours, minutes . . . or seconds, as we have mentioned. It all depends on how aligned the various levels are, through our U-Flow, which we will be returning to shortly, along with a DW/ DW exercise.

Focus On What You Want

There seems to be a general rule in life based around the idea that we tend to get more of what we focus on. But when many of us are seeking to change something, we tend to focus on that *thing we want to change* even more, which seems to perpetuate it. In other words, the more we focus on what we don't want, the more we seem to get it.

To help with this, consider an idea that says our subconscious mind filters out the negative words in statements like these:

- I want to stop binge eating.
- I want to stop lying awake at night.
- I want to stop thinking that dogs or bees will hurt me.

So, subconsciously, we filter out the word 'stop' so the emphasis is on . . .

- . . . binge eating
- . . . lying awake at night
- . . . dogs or bees hurting me

If we can switch our focus from what we *don't* want to a *positively phrased version* of what we *do* want, and put our energy into that, we are likely to get far better results.

- . . . eat normally
- . . . sleep deeply
- . . . feel safe around dogs and bees

If focusing on what we want is the aim, then why bother with the 'Don't Want/Do Want' – why not just the 'Do Want'?

Well, there's a weird phenomenon I noticed by accident, really, which I'll come on to shortly, but the spoiler alert now is that very often we need the 'Don't Want' to make the 'Do Want' more effective!

To help clarify, let's see if we can apply what we have learned so far to something we actually want to change now.

Think way back to Exercise 3, 'Your Wishlist', and your 3-2-1 analysis of those three main categories of your life: Health and Well-being, Career and Money, Relationships and Intimacy. In each of these areas that you want to change, there is something about the way that you are thinking, feeling or behaving that is creating an effect, an outcome or results that you do not want in your life. You want to stop or reduce that happening and start or increase something else instead. There is something that you don't want – the old surface-level symptoms – and there is something that you do want – a new, more desirable positive outcome – which we can summarize as a Don't Want/Do Want (DW/DW) statement:

- I don't want [. . .], I do want [. . .] instead.

First we are going to apply this at surface level – then we shall dig a little deeper.

Exercise 19: Health and Well-being Don't Want/Do Want

Duration: 20–30 minutes
Journal Required: Yes
Buddy Required: Optional but can be helpful

Background

If we can take a surface-level symptom that we don't want and identify an opposite, positively phrased version of a desired outcome that we do want, and focus our conscious mind there, it can send a powerful message to our subconscious mind to help bring about a transformation in these areas.

Instructions

Part 1

1. On a new page in your journal, write the heading 'Health and Well-being Don't Want/Do Want'.
2. Divide the page into three columns and add the labels, as shown below. Ignore the middle column for now, but make sure it is there.

DON'T WANT		DO WANT

3. Look back in your journal at the 3-2-1 analysis you did on Health and Well-being in Exercise 3 'Your Wishlist' and write the two things you would like to change and one thing that you feel needs to change in the 'Don't Want' column, in the form of something you no longer want. There may be just one phrase for each or you may find several come to mind, but keep it focused on that one topic area for now. *Focus is important.* For example, two things you would like to change could be:

- I don't want to feel achy, sluggish and unfit in the morning.
- When busy, I don't want to get by, eating things that I know are not good for me and make me feel uncomfortable afterwards.

One thing that needs to change could be:

- I don't want to fit in my health around everything else and it to always be last on my list.

NOTE: Doing this in your head will not work nearly as well – you will need to write it down for maximum benefit.

4. For each and every 'negative' statement, underline the negative word and create an equal and opposite 'positive' statement, writing it down in the 'Do Want' column. You may find that other ideas come to mind as you do this.

DON'T WANT		DO WANT
I don't want to feel <u>achy</u>, <u>sluggish</u> and <u>unfit in the morning</u>.		In the morning I want to wake feeling able to <u>move freely</u>, full of <u>energy</u> and <u>fit</u> to take on the day.
When busy, I don't want to <u>get by</u>, eating things that I know are <u>not good for me and make me feel uncomfortable afterwards</u>.		Even when busy, I want to <u>take time</u> to make sure I eat things that are <u>good for me and give me a good, nourished feeling afterwards</u>.
I don't want to <u>fit in my health</u> around everything else and it always be <u>last on my list</u>.		I want to make <u>health my priority</u>, and fit in the rest of my life around it.

5. Go through your 'Do Want' list and make sure there are no negative words, i.e. you cannot say, 'Don't Want = Stressed, Do Want = *Not* Stressed'. You must find the *opposite, positive* version of the negative words or phrase, even if there is resistance. In fact, especially if there is resistance! For example, 'Don't Want = Stressed, Do Want = Calm and Relaxed'. Get help from an opposites (antonyms) dictionary or an E.S.C.A.P.E. Buddy for ideas, but it must be your word(s) you choose, not someone else's.
6. Read through your list of positive 'I wants' noticing anything you feel as you do so. They should feel good and inspirational to read!

NOTE: Doing this goes against a lot of positive-thinking-type books and teachings that state it is wrong to say 'I want'. What I have noticed is that saying what you WANT is actually like a stepping stone, taking you one step closer towards the goal, but much less likely to trigger resistance.

If we phrased them like typical affirmations –

- I focus on my health
- I am fit
- I eat well
- I sleep well
- I awaken energized

– the critical faculty is likely to trigger resistance at this early stage, with that little voice at the back of your mind saying 'Oh really?' But keeping it as something you want first of all will usually lower that resistance and *allow the idea past your critical faculty and into your subconscious.*

Later in your journey, once you get more familiar with the new ideas, you can then switch to a more traditional affirmative version as it will begin to feel more truthful.

7. As you read through the 'Do Want' list, check for any resistance or discomfort, however, and if you notice any, ask yourself why and make a separate note in your journal. We may need to dig a little deeper, but it may also be that you simply need to find a different word or phrase that feels better.

8. Now, go through your list in a different way, first reading the negative, then the positive, like this:

- I don't want to feel achy, sluggish and unfit in the morning, I want to wake feeling able to move freely, full of energy and fit to take on the day.
- When busy, I don't want to get by eating things that I know are not good for me and make me feel uncomfortable afterwards, I want to take time to make sure I eat things that are good for me and make me feel good and nourished afterwards.
- I don't want to fit in my health around everything else and it always be last on my list, I want to make health my priority, and fit in the rest of my life around it.

Again, contrary to what I have read in many positive-thinking-type books, I find that often when working with clients it actually helps to do some *deliberate negative thinking*, verbalizing the negative and even repeating it, before we aim for the positive.

Many people fear it will reinforce the negative, but if you say the negative first, it actually helps to release it and ease the pressure in some way.

By acknowledging the negative and then focusing on the positive, we are helping to bring thoughts and ideas that would otherwise go unchallenged into our conscious awareness and so interrupting the continual reconditioning and rehypnotizing that would otherwise happen.

With a client I will sometimes get them to verbalize the negative numerous times, especially if there is emotion attached, as each time they say it, some of the suppressed or repressed emotion may be released. Then when I feel the emotion is reducing, I will get them to add on the positive as well. With the critical faculty softened by the verbalization of the negatives, the positive ideas have more 'space' to take root.

Ultimately, the aim is to no longer need to state the negative, so that we are just left with a more positive, affirmative version, which then becomes our new mantra or self-talk and helps form our new identity. But trying to be too positive, too quickly, can rapidly backfire and actually have a negative effect. Stating the negative first reduces this effect and enhances the positive.

Part 2 – Convert the 'One Thing' to an Identity Statement

To do this we simply take a phrase like a Don't Want/Do Want and reword it into more of a generalization about who we are or who we want to be as a person. Again, using both sides of the DW/DW works well to begin with.

> **I don't want to be someone who [old Don't Want], I want to be someone who [new Do Want].**

That 'one thing' that needs to change will very often underpin or lay the foundation for enabling the other 'two things' we'd *like* to change as well, so we'll use this to create an Identity Statement for this exercise, but feel free to choose one of the others if it seems a better fit.

I don't want to be someone who fits in health around everything else, with it always being last on my list, I want to be some-one who makes health my priority and fits in the rest of my life around it.

Part 3 – Create a Health and Well-being Summary Statement

What we need to do now is create a summary statement that encompasses *all* of these ideas. This will enable us to:

- Acknowledge and reinforce our current positives, while bringing the current negatives into awareness for examination.
- Lay the foundation for a deep and lasting transformation by initiating an Identity Switch.
- Have some specific, practical ideas or behaviours we can focus on and put into practice immediately, *today*, to help make the new way become a part of everyday life.

In so doing, we deprogramme ourselves from what has gone before and give our subconscious inner librarian a new set of inner references for what to think and how to be in certain situations; we also help our brains adapt to and support the change by encouraging Hebbian Learning – this time consciously, working in our favour, rather than subconsciously, which we have previously had to fight against.

The general formula for the summary statement will go something like:

In the area of health and well-being, I [insert positive 1, 2 and 3 from your 3-2-1 'Wishlist' exercise]. However, from now on, I [insert your old/new DW/DW Identity Statement], which means that I [insert your DW/DW 'two things']. I am committed to doing this now because [think about your 'why' and relate it to one or more of the core beliefs].

An example could be:

In the area of health and well-being, I am reasonably healthy, knowledgeable about what I am supposed to do and able to be disciplined when I really feel like it. However, from now on, I don't want to be someone who fits in health around everything else, with it always being last on my list. I want to be someone who makes health my priority and fits in the rest of my life around it.

I don't want to feel achy, sluggish and unfit in the morning, I want to wake feeling able to move freely, full of energy and fit to take on the day.

When busy, I don't want to get by eating things that I know are not good for me and make me feel uncomfortable afterwards, I want to take time to make sure I eat things that are good for me and make me feel good and nourished afterwards.

I am committed to this more than ever now because it will help me to feel good about myself, more in control of my health and well-being along with a greater sense of peace as I go to bed each night.

(I know this is long, repetitive and may require you to write out similar statements numerous times . . . but each time you do, with focus and attention, you are undoing the thousands of times you have previously focused on the old, negative opposite, and paving the way for something new.)

This summary statement should feel good when you read it, both to yourself and out loud. Treat it like a medical prescription to be taken twice a day, once in the morning and once in the evening, topped up in between as opportunities arise, for at least a week to ten days, or until no longer required.

I know it is not exactly your typical short and snappy 'I am worthy' type of mantra, but if carried out with honesty and attention to detail it should hit home much more deeply.

Providing it is accepted, we have a big enough 'Why' and we are more 'committed' than 'interested', repetition and focus on this new idea or ideas will then help to trigger the behaviours that go with them, such as eating better, exercising more regularly, prioritizing daily schedules, sleeping better and so on.

NOTE: Throughout your day, any time you feel any negative thoughts arising around the topic of Health and Well-being, first see if you can identify which of the negative thoughts it is. Then, instead of trying to ignore it, actually verbalize or state the old 'Don't Want' to yourself, first, like a negative mantra, and *then* remind yourself of the opposite, positive version that you do want. If a negative thought comes to mind that is not on your list, add it in and repeat the process.

Resistance

If you feel any resistance anywhere, that is OK. Stay focused on the exercise and repeat it as best you can. Sometimes we need persistence, remember, but we will also deal with any resistance shortly, as well as explaining what that middle column is for.

For now, though, take a break, and let's repeat the whole exercise for those other two areas, Career and Money, and Relationships and Intimacy.

Exercise 20: Career and Money
Don't Want/Do Want

Duration: 20–30 minutes
Journal Required: Yes
Buddy Required: Optional but can be helpful

Background

If we can take surface-level symptoms relating to Career and Money and create opposite, positively phrased versions of more desirable outcomes, and focus our conscious mind there, it can send a powerful message to our subconscious mind to help bring about transformations in these areas.

Instructions

Part 1

1. On a new page in your journal, write the heading 'Career and Wealth Don't Want/Do Want'.
2. Divide the page into three columns and add the 'Don't Want' and 'Do Want' labels as in the previous exercise.
3. Look back in your journal at the 3-2-1 analysis you did on Career and Money in the 'Wishlist' exercise. Write the two things you would like to change and the one thing you feel needs to change in the 'Don't Want' column, in the form of something you no longer want. For example, two things you would like to change could be:

- I don't want to have to work evenings and weekends, when everyone else is having fun.
- I don't want to have to take on work I no longer enjoy, just to pay the bills.

One thing that needs to change could be:

- I don't want to just 'get by' any more, only earning enough to furnish debts and expenses, with little left over.

4. For each and every 'negative' statement, underline the negative words and create an equal and opposite 'positive' statement, writing it down in the 'Do Want' column. You may find that other ideas come to mind as you do this.

DON'T WANT		DO WANT
I don't want to have to <u>work evenings</u> and <u>weekends</u>, when <u>everyone else is having fun</u>.		I want my <u>evenings and weekends to be free</u>, so I can <u>have fun with my friends or family</u>.
I don't want to have to <u>take on work I no longer enjoy</u>, that I feel I have to, just to <u>pay the bills</u>.		I want to focus on <u>what I enjoy</u>, that I <u>want</u> to do, that I can <u>put my heart into</u> because <u>I love to do it</u> and am good at it.
I don't want to just <u>'get by'</u> any more, only earning <u>enough to furnish debts and expenses</u>, with <u>little left over</u>.		I want to <u>financially thrive</u>, be <u>in credit everywhere</u>, with <u>surplus funds</u> to do what I want with.

5. Again, go through your 'Do Want' list and make sure there are no negative words. Remember, you cannot say, 'Don't Want = Boring Job, Do Want = *Not* Boring Job'. You must force your

mind to find an *opposite, positive* version of the negative words or phrase, especially if there is resistance! For example, 'Don't Want = Boring Job, Do Want = Interesting Job'.

6. Read through your list of positive 'I wants', noticing anything you feel as you do so. They should feel good to read!

7. As you read through the 'Do Want' list, check for any resistance or discomfort, however, and if you notice any, ask yourself why and make a separate note in your journal. Again, we may need to dig a little deeper, but it may also be that you simply need to find a different word or phrase that feels better.

8. Now, as before, go through this list again, first reading the negative, then the positive, as follows:

- I don't want to have to work evenings and weekends, when everyone else is having fun. I want my evenings and weekends to be free, so I can have fun with my friends or family.
- I don't want to have to take on work I no longer enjoy, that I feel I have to, just to pay the bills. I want to focus on what I enjoy, that I want to do, that I can put my heart into because I love to do it and am good at it.
- I don't want to just 'get by' any more, only earning enough to furnish debts and expenses, with little left over. I want to financially thrive, be in credit everywhere, with surplus funds to do what I want with.

Remember that by acknowledging the negative and then focusing on the positive, we are helping to bring thoughts and ideas that would otherwise go unchallenged into our conscious awareness, which helps to interrupt the subconscious processes that would happen otherwise, and so dissolve resistance to the new ideas.

Part 2 – Convert the 'One Thing' to an Identity Statement

To do this we simply take the 'one thing' Don't Want/Do Want and reword it into more of a generalization about who we are or who we want to be as a person. Again, using both sides of the DW/DW works well to begin with, and feel free to swap out for one of the others if need be, but try the 'one thing' phrase first.

> *I don't want to be someone who [old Don't Want], I want to be someone who [new Do Want].*

For example:

> *I don't want to be someone who just 'gets by' any more, only earning enough to furnish debts and expenses, with little left over. I want to be someone who financially thrives, is in credit everywhere, with surplus funds to do what I want with.*

That new Identity Statement should feel good and begin to spark ideas inside about what needs to happen to make that more of a reality. Your current situation would have been created or formed as outcomes from your old beliefs and identity-driven behaviours, over a period of time. As you focus on this new idea now, we are beginning to slow that old 'down' escalator so that it can eventually stop, change direction and become an 'up' one, taking you more in the direction you want.

Part 3 – Create a Career and Money Summary Statement

Refer back to the previous exercise if you need clarification, but remember, the general formula is . . .

> *In the area of Career and Money, I [insert positive 1, 2 and 3 from your 3-2-1 'Wishlist' exercise]. However, from now on I [insert your old/new DW/DW Identity Statement], which means that I [insert your DW/DW 'two things']. I am committed to doing this*

now because *[think about your 'why' and relate it to one or more of the core beliefs].*

An example could be:

In the area of Career and Money, I am good at creating opportunities, willing to work hard when necessary, and always aim to do a really good job of whatever I do. However, I no longer want to be someone who just 'gets by', only earning enough to furnish debts and expenses, with little left over. I want to be someone who financially thrives, is in credit everywhere, with surplus funds to do what I want with.

I don't want to have to take on work I no longer enjoy, that I feel I have to, just to pay the bills. I want to focus on what I enjoy, that I want to do, that I can put my heart into because I love to do it and am good at it.

I don't want to have to work evenings and weekends, when everyone else is having fun. I want my evenings and weekends to be free, so I can have fun with my friends or family.

I am committed to doing this because it will help me feel really good about myself, as well as lighter and freer.

Again, treat it like a medical prescription to be taken twice a day, once in the morning and once in the evening, topped up in between as opportunities arise, for at least a week to ten days, or until no longer required!

Read it aloud, let the thoughts and words become a part of your self-talk. You are dehypnotizing from the old and educating your subconscious as to what kind of experiences you would like to bring into life instead. You still have to make the choices and actions to allow this to happen as a physical experience, but the more your mind focuses on these new ideas, unchallenged, the more your inner mind can go to work for you, in the same way it always has – only this time with more conscious direction and awareness.

NOTE: Throughout your day, any time you feel any negative thoughts arising around the topic of Career and Money, see if you can identify which of the negative thoughts it is, and remind yourself of the opposite that you do want. If it is not on your list, add it in and repeat the process above.

Resistance

If you feel any resistance anywhere, that is OK. Stay focused on the exercise and repeat it as best you can. We will deal with any resistance shortly, when we understand what the middle column is for.

For now, though, take a break, and let's repeat the whole exercise for Relationships and Intimacy.

Exercise 21: Relationships and Intimacy Don't Want/Do Want

Duration: 20–30 minutes
Journal Required: Yes
Buddy Required: Optional but can be helpful

Background

If we can identify your 'Don't Wants' and 'Do Wants' relating to Relationships and Intimacy, and send a powerful message to both your conscious and subconscious mind to help bring about changes in these areas, your life will be filled with a greater sense of happiness, satisfaction and enjoyment, which will provide a foundation for the same in other areas of your life.

Instructions

Part 1

1. On a new page in your journal, write the heading 'Relationships and Intimacy Don't Want/Do Want'.
2. Divide the page into three columns and add the 'Don't Want' and 'Do Want' labels as in the previous exercises.
3. Look back in your journal at the 3-2-1 analysis you did on Relationships and Intimacy in the 'Wishlist' exercise. Write the two things you would like to change and one thing that you feel needs to change in the 'Don't Want' column, in the form of something you no longer want. For example, two things you might want to change could be:

   - I don't want to feel uncomfortable and anxious around social situations any more, having to hold myself back, afraid of saying what I think.
   - I don't want to put my friends and family at the bottom of the list, only able to relax and have fun with them when I have completed everything else.

   One thing that needs to change could be:

   - I want to stop putting up a protective barrier between myself and others, scared to fully engage, which means I never get as close as I could.

4. For each and every 'negative' statement, underline the negative words and create an equal and opposite positive statement, writing it down in the 'Do Want' column.

DON'T WANT		DO WANT
I don't want to feel <u>uncomfortable</u> and <u>anxious</u> around social situations, having to <u>hold myself back</u>, <u>afraid of saying what I think</u>.		I want to feel <u>comfortable</u> and <u>relaxed</u> around social situations, <u>able to let go</u> and <u>be myself</u>, <u>happy to say what I think</u>.
I don't want to put my friends and family at the <u>bottom of the list</u>, only able to relax and have fun with them <u>when</u> I have <u>completed everything else</u>.		I want to make time with friends and family as <u>important as anything else</u>, an equal priority I plan and allow for, <u>irrespective of what else I have on</u>.
I want to stop <u>putting up a protective barrier</u> between myself and others, <u>scared to fully engage</u>, which means I <u>never get as close as I could</u>.		I want to be more <u>open</u> and more <u>willing to engage</u> with others, so that I can <u>feel closer</u> and have <u>more meaningful relationships</u>.

5. Again, go through your 'Do Want' list and make sure there are no negative words. Remember, you cannot say, 'Don't Want = Arguments, Do Want = *No* Arguments'. You must force your mind to find an *opposite*, *positive* version of the negative words or phrase, especially if there is resistance! For example: 'Don't Want = Arguments, Do Want = Discussions or Agreements'.

6. Read through your list of positive 'I wants', noticing anything you feel as you do so. They should feel good to read!

7. As you read through the 'Do Want' list, check for any resistance or discomfort, however, and if you notice any, ask yourself why and make a separate note in your journal. Again, we may need to dig a little deeper, but it may also be that you simply need to find a different word or phrase that feels better.

8. Now, go through your list, as with the others, first reading the negative, then the positive, as follows:

- I don't want to feel uncomfortable and anxious around social situations, having to hold myself back, afraid of saying what I think. I want to feel comfortable and relaxed around social situations, able to let go and be myself, happy to say what I think.
- I don't want to put my friends and family at the bottom of the list, only able to relax and have fun with them when I have completed everything else. I want to make time with friends and family as important as anything else, an equal priority I plan and allow for, irrespective of what else I have on.
- I want to stop putting up a protective barrier between myself and others, scared to fully engage, which means I never get as close as I could. I want to be more open and more willing to engage with others, so that I can feel closer and have even more meaningful relationships.

Part 2 – Convert the 'One Thing' to an Identity Statement

As before, simply take the 'one thing' Don't Want/Do Want and reword it into more of a generalization about who we are or who we want to be as a person. Again, using both sides of the DW/DW works well to begin with, and feel free to swap out for one of the others if need be, but try the 'one thing' phrase first.

> *I don't want to be someone who [old Don't Want], I want to be someone who [new Do Want].*

For example:

> *I no longer want to be someone who puts up a protective barrier between myself and others, scared to fully engage, so that I never*

*get as close as I could. I want to be someone who is open and
willing to engage with others, so that I can feel closer and have
even more meaningful relationships.*

That new Identity Statement can then trigger the behaviours
and actions to help bring that about. BUT . . . we cannot demand
things of others if we are not willing to give it ourselves. If we want
love, we must be loving; if we want to feel cared for, we must also
show care; if we want to be ourselves, we must also allow others
to be themselves (provided no harmful boundaries are crossed, of
course).

Part 3 – Create a Relationships and Intimacy Summary Statement

Refer back to the previous exercise if you need clarification, but
remember, the general formula is . . .

> *In the area of Relationships and Intimacy, I [insert positive 1, 2
> and 3 from your 3-2-1 'Wishlist' exercise]. However, from now on I
> [insert your old/new DW/DW Identity Statement], which means
> that I [insert your DW/DW 'two things']. I am committed to
> doing this now because [think about your 'why' and relate it to one
> or more of the core beliefs].*

An example could be:

> *In the area of Relationships and Intimacy, I am friendly,
> thoughtful and kind. However, I no longer want to be someone
> who puts up a protective barrier between myself and others, scared
> to fully engage, so that I never get as close as I could. I want to be
> someone who is open and willing to engage with others, so that I
> can feel closer and have even more meaningful relationships.*
>   *I don't want to put my friends and family at the bottom of
> the list, only able to relax and have fun with them when I have
> completed everything else. I want to make time with friends and*

family as important as anything else, an equal priority I plan and allow for, irrespective of what else I have on.

I don't want to feel uncomfortable and anxious around social situations, having to hold myself back, afraid of saying what I think. I want to feel comfortable and relaxed around social situations, able to let go and be myself, happy to say what I think.

I am committed to doing this because it will help me feel really good about myself, more secure in personal and social situations, in control without being controlling, more accepted, with more fun and more pleasure, as well as feeling lighter and freer.

Again, this should feel good when you read it and, again, treat it like a medical prescription, once in the morning and once in the evening, topped up in between as opportunities arise, for at least a week to ten days, or until no longer required!

Ideally, the Identity Statement should pave the way or lay the foundation to facilitate the other, more specific areas, provided we follow it through with actions in alignment with this.

NOTE: Throughout your day, any time you feel any negative thoughts arising around the topic of Relationships and Intimacy, see if you can identify which of the negative thoughts it is and remind yourself of the opposite that you do want. If it is not on your list, add it in and update your list, as before.

Resistance

If you feel any resistance anywhere, that is OK. Stay focused on the exercise and repeat it as best you can. For now, though, take a break, and then we'll explore how to deepen the effect.

Mind the Gap

The 'Don't Want/Do Want' exercise is a great place to start to begin switching your thoughts and behaviours to more positive outcomes. If you can get a positive result that way, great, we are moving from the down side of the U-Flow to the up, and that area of your life can begin to change.

But what if there is still resistance? I always set the initial DW/DW exercise for my students, asking them to think about an area they would like to work on, chat through it with each other and create a DW/DW list. But I began to notice something when wandering around the classroom peeking in on them practising. They would often be chatting away about something entirely unrelated to the exercise, telling me how they'd finished it in five minutes and were just passing time.

But when I looked closer, they had barely scratched the surface. After asking each other to write down their 'Don't Wants' and convert them to 'Do Wants', I noticed they had often done one of two things. They had either:

1. Kept it so surface level, or generic, it really did not create any inner feeling for change, OR
2. They had completely skipped a level in some way and their 'Do Wants' and 'Don't Wants' just didn't match up – again, keeping it quite surface level.

Interestingly, the bit they had skipped was nearly always where *the real transformation needed to take place*. They were subconsciously resisting – invisible beliefs were influencing their behaviour and a subtle form of the threat response was causing them to keep things very surface level – at the top of our U-Flow system – when actually the real magic needed to occur a level or two deeper. Or they were avoiding the REAL want, and so jumping to something else, a step ahead.

Think of it this way. When there are simple opposites, with no emotional significance attached, there will usually be little or no resistance to change. A person who is cold may want to be warm or hot. A person who is wet may want to be dry.

DON'T WANT	DO WANT
Cold	Warm
Wet	Dry

But if we bring in personal, emotional, habitual and behavioural problems, threat response induced anomalies can begin to appear. Let's use the example of weight loss, an area of concern and frustration for millions of people.

If I ask someone to do the DW/DW exercise around weight loss, and say OK, tell me what you want, the usual answer is 'to lose weight'.

But if the person has been struggling to lose weight until now, there will be a reason or reasons. It's actually not that difficult to lose weight, under the right conditions. After being captured at Dunkirk during the Second World War while defending a bridge to allow fellow soldiers to retreat to the beaches, spending four years in a concentration camp and then finally enduring three months of the 'Death Marches' at the end of the war, surviving on grass, bugs and any scraps he could find, my grandfather lost weight easily, becoming little more than a walking skeleton by the time he was finally liberated. He didn't want to lose weight, but the conditions made it easy for him to do so.

This may be an extreme example, and I am in no way suggesting that course of action, but the same is true for anybody with a weight condition – losing weight itself is not actually difficult. However, *creating the right conditions to do so* often is, especially with so many influences nowadays.

Leaving aside genetics, microbiome and other physiological factors (which we will look into in Part Three), if we want to lose weight or create any kind of transformation in life, instead of focusing on the result itself it is often much more effective to focus on *creating the right conditions* to do so – just as we saw in the Izzy and Kate case studies. Once we do this, everything else very often takes care of itself.

One of the aims of the DW/DW is to help achieve that, but very often we have internal resistance to creating those conditions and that is what we are interested in here. Walking around the classroom, I often noticed it was the 'gap' or the bit that students were skipping that held the key to creating the right conditions. If you found any resistance in the previous DW/DW exercises, it is probably this gap we need to take a closer look at now.

Conflicting Ideas and Secondary Gains

When there is something we want to change, it's amazing how reluctant we can be to voice the positive outcome we want if it is outside of our accepted belief system to have it. Staying with the weight loss example, while most people are happy to say that they want to lose weight, many will find it difficult to actually say, 'I want to be slim'; and even more difficult to elaborate further, such as feeling more attractive or more sexy, for example, if that is applicable.

When this happens, however subtly, it is a sign of resistance to change and we must become aware of this and resolve it if we are to be successful.

Sometimes this will be a very mild discomfort at first which, once expressed, becomes acceptable very quickly. Other times, though, there will be much greater resistance – which is fear, remember – creating conflicting ideas that will cause problems.

The easiest way to explain this is to use an example, and I'll stay with this weight loss one for now, though the principles apply to any area of life.

Let's say we ask someone who wants to lose weight to complete the DW/DW.

DON'T WANT	DO WANT
I don't want to be fat and overweight.	I want to be slim and healthy.

Sounds great, and this is the point I see many of my students get to when they think they are top of the class for getting it done so quickly. But when I see this, or the equivalent, I always ask them to dig deeper on each side of the statement, usually with a simple question such as 'What's that like?' and then 'Where does that leave you, what outcome?' And here is where it starts to get interesting.

ME: Being, or feeling, fat and overweight, what's that like?
CLIENT: I feel low self-worth.
ME: And where does that leave you?
CLIENT: Feeling unattractive . . . but safe!
ME: Ah, OK. And the opposite, being slim, what's *that* like?
CLIENT: I feel good about myself.
ME: And where does that leave you, what outcomes?
CLIENT: Feeling more attractive . . . but scary!

Can you see the problem? By digging deeper we unravel more of the resistance and our DW/DW actually becomes . . .

DON'T WANT	DO WANT
I don't want to be overweight.	I do want to be slim.
What's that like? Low self-worth	*What's that like?* Feeling good about myself
Where does that leave you? Feeling unattractive (but I do feel **safe**)	*Where does that leave you?* Feeling attractive (but feeling **unsafe**)

By asking a question and facing up to the honest answer, we are suddenly aware of our invisible beliefs and subconscious conflicts. In this example, if we attempt to lose weight we are also attempting to move from feeling safe to feeling unsafe – which is hardly motivating and will make us highly prone to behaviours that will seem like self-sabotage on the surface but are actually subconscious threat responses helping to 'protect' us.

Although, on the surface, staying overweight may be causing us problems, underneath it is actually helping us to achieve something. When this happens we call it a 'secondary gain'.

To stand any chance of a successful change in this area we need to remove the need for the secondary gain. And, by the way, have you noticed how the conflict and secondary gain involves one of our core beliefs around safeness, feeling safe and secure in the world?

There could be any number of reasons why we may feel unsafe feeling slim and attractive, for example, but they will all involve some kind of life experience or thing we have learned that has caused us to think and feel that way. And so we could now begin to dig deeper still and explore those memories and life experiences, as we have done with other examples, to help understand and undo the origins.

We don't always need to but, for the sake of this example, let's say we originally experienced some kind of trauma or incident that made us feel that being 'slim and attractive' was not safe. Perhaps we felt helpless, powerless, out of control and unable to say no to someone or something, and this caused us such anxiety that it has stayed with us ever since, the threat response causing us to do whatever it takes to never feel that way again.

But as we re-evaluate now, let go of any suppressed or repressed emotions and begin to feel and see any such incidents from a new perspective, we realize that we are an adult now, stronger, more powerful and able to exercise choice, saying no to things that will cause us harm and yes to things that will be good for us.

All this can lead us to form a new idea, a new belief: 'It is safe for me to be slim now.'

Remember, it is the belief that is important, not necessarily what caused it. Exploring memories, especially with regression, in hypnosis is an amazing tool for doing this, but it is a means to an end, not the end itself. What we really need to happen is to form new ideas that support the new desired outcome.

How do we create the right conditions so that we can lose weight? In this example we obviously need to accept that it is indeed *safe* for us to do so!

So very often, in the middle of the Don't Want/Do Want, there will be a gap – something we *really* want (or even *need*) in order to achieve the thing we originally wanted. And, surprise, surprise, the gap in the middle will nearly always involve a core belief.

DON'T WANT	REAL DO WANT	OUTCOME
Overweight	Feel SAFE being slim	Slim
Low self-worth		Good about self
Feel unattractive		Feel attractive
But safe		Feel safe

Previously, 'I don't want to be overweight, I want to be slim' would have created conflict – resistance. But if we can now focus on the idea of it feeling *safe* to be slim, we are more likely to follow through with the actions required to bring about the original desired outcome.

We can also then add in some specifics that both support the new core idea and lead on from it, which we can use as autosuggestions, mantras or *real* affirmations. These are sometimes 'which means that' statements:

It is safe for me to be slim now, which means that I can create the right conditions to do so now.

DON'T WANT	NEW BELIEFS	WHICH MEANS THAT
Overweight Low self-worth Feel unattractive But safe	It is safe for me to feel slim and attractive, because I am an adult now and can say no if I need to.	I can eat more healthily, do more exercise, feel attractive and good about myself and that's OK.

If we were to repeat the statements in the 'new beliefs' and 'which means that' columns to ourselves, and could accept them, we would begin to notice a much more profound change than when we were just scraping the surface.

If we were to generalize, we could put it like this:

DON'T WANT	REAL WANT/NEED	WHICH MEANS THAT
The surface-level symptoms, original issue and what it currently means to us.	The beliefs that will allow us to FEEL different and thereby create the right conditions – usually core beliefs.	We can now have, do or be what we *need* to give us what we wanted in the first place.

If you experienced any resistance in any of the previous exercises, it probably means we need to drop down a level and fill in the gap in the DW/DW exercises. To do this, we use a process I call Three Levels Deep.

Three Levels Deep

When working one-to-one with a client, to help them release the brakes or move on in some area of their life, I would rarely take things at face value. Instead, I would nearly always drop down at least a level or two of the U-Flow before aiming to help them turn things around. But students would often ask me, 'How do you know how far to go? How do you know when you have hit the root of an issue?'

I would usually answer by saying that I keep going until I hit one or more core beliefs, and then begin to turn things around from there, but to make things simpler and give more of a structure to follow, I created the 'Three Levels Deep' exercise.

The aim is to help the client – in this case you – be able to express their problem in three levels, rather like a mini U-Flow.

The three levels are:

Level 1 – What's the current situation?
Level 2 – What's that like for you?
Level 3 – Where does that leave you?

Each question, answered honestly, should take you a level deeper in your mind and actually reveal more of the automatic, subconscious processes that have been influencing how you have been thinking, feeling and behaving, often without fully recognizing it.

Remember, the deeper the level at which we can bring about change, the more profound and lasting the eventual surface-level transformation. So if we do the 'Three Levels Deep' exercise, and apply the DW/DW to the lowest level first, and then work our way back up, we often get a more profound transformation than if we had stayed purely at the surface.

Very often, the surface-level ideas can seem very complex, but the deeper we go, the simpler they become; and – if answered honestly – the more they can hit home.

You can apply this 'Three Levels Deep' exercise to any area of life or anywhere you experience resistance, but for illustration purposes here we are going to use it on the DW/DW 'Wishlist' exercises for the three main areas of life we have been exploring to see what else comes up.

Exercise 22: Going Three Levels Deep

Duration: 15–20 minutes
Journal Required: Yes
Buddy Required: Not essential but can be very helpful

Background

If you have carried out the DW/DW exercise but are still experiencing a sense of resistance, it is usually beneficial to dig a little deeper into what is going on, and the 'Three Levels Deep' exercise is a simple but effective way to garner more information and insight.

You can apply this to any area of life really but for the purposes of this exercise we are going to apply it to the 'one thing' that needs to change, from each area of your original '3-2-1 Wishlist' analysis on Health and Well-being, Career and Money, and Relationships and Intimacy.

Instructions

Part 1

On a new page in your journal, write the heading 'Three Levels Deep Exercise on Health and Well-being'. Think about the one thing you feel needs to change in relation to your health and well-being, and draw a table like the one below, filling most of the page to ensure there is plenty of space.

	OLD	NEW
Current situation		
What's that like?		
Where does that leave you? What outcome?		

In the top box of the left-hand column, write down your 'one thing' that needs to change relating to Health and Well-being in the form of something you are currently doing. Continuing our example from earlier, this would be: 'Fitting in my health around everything else and it always being last on my list.'

Then ask yourself, 'What's that like, doing that?' and take a moment to really think about it. Think about what it feels like to be you, living that current situation, noticing any feelings or emotions that arise as you do. Write the answer in the box underneath. For example: 'Like I am always behind, struggling to keep up, out of control.'

Finally, think about the question, 'Where does that leave you? What's the overall outcome of that?' and write the answer in the bottom left box. For example: 'A bit lost, feeling not good enough, like I've failed in some way.'

It should look something like this:

	OLD	NEW
Current situation	Fitting in my health around everything else and it always being last on my list.	
What's that like?	Like I am always behind, struggling to keep up, **out of control.**	
Where does that leave you? What outcome?	A bit lost, feeling **not good enough**, like I've failed in some way.	

Can you spot the core beliefs that get pushed to the surface? Out of control and 'not enoughness'?

What if we could now apply the DW/DW to this *bottom level*, and let go of any ideas of 'not enoughness'? What if we could also apply the 'Awareness of Meaning' exercise and 'Increasing Your Sense of "Enoughness"' exercise to this level as well?

Could we, for a moment, slow down, pause, stop, take a breath, interrupt the usual response of attaching negative meanings, beating ourselves up and trying to run even faster up that down escalator? Could we instead just sit with any feelings that arise and let them pass, gently?

Could we be willing to consider that the Real You, the one underneath all the fears and limitations, is enough anyway, simply by existing? Could we allow ourselves to feel good enough anyway, even though we haven't yet achieved what we want to? Could we be willing to release any judgement and accept ourselves as we are? We may not like the situation, but could we at least stop judging ourselves for it, which only rehypnotizes and reconditions, keeping us stuck in a loop? Could we tell that inner security system to stand down, chill out, relax, so that we can regain a sense of worth and control?

Because if we can, we can begin to take action from a much better place. Remember, whatever feeling drives a behaviour will, ultimately, probably just create more of the same feeling. If we can begin to accept our sense of worth and value, our 'enoughness', as being innate, indestructible, unquestionable, we can take a solid step across our Three Levels Deep mini U-Flow and create a new Level 3, which can provide a more solid foundation that will help us move more steadily up the other side.

Now, when we ask 'What's *that* like?' in relation to the new core belief feeling of 'enoughness' in the new Level 3, we might find that we feel safer, more secure, more in control and more on top of things, which forms our new Level 2. And if we ask 'What does that mean, now?', in relation to where we started, it means that we can now *really and more easily* focus on making health a priority, creating a new, better current situation or 'more desirable outcome' (from our main U-Flow) that we wanted all along.

	OLD	NEW
Current situation	Fitting in my health around everything else and it always being last on my list.	Making health my priority, and fitting in the rest of my life around it.
What's that like?	Like I am always behind, struggling to keep up, **out of control.**	I can feel safe, secure, on top of things and more in control.

Where does that leave you? What outcome?	A bit lost, feeling **not good enough**, like I've failed in some way.	I am good enough, right here, right now, exactly as I am.

And if we refer back to our Health and Well-being summary statement, now, instead of doing all that because it will give us something – our 'why' – we can discover that the thing we wanted – a sense of 'enoughness' – was actually there within us all along. The difference now is that instead of it being the 'outcome' we are chasing, it is the driving force for change, coming from within us. Instead of chasing the outer world to create a different inner world, focusing on a different inner world – the Real You – will help to create a new outer one.

We can transpose this into our Health and Well-being summary statement, maybe even dropping the negatives now.

In the example we have been using, our summary statement can now become this:

In the area of health and well-being, I have been reasonably healthy, knowledgeable about what I am supposed to do, and able to be disciplined when I really feel like it.

However, from now on, I want to remember my innate worth and value even more, my unquestionable sense of 'enoughness', exactly as I am, right here, right now, because the more I accept this, the better I feel and the more in control I feel.

As a result, the more I am becoming someone who makes health my priority and fits in the rest of my life around it now.

Each morning, I can begin to wake feeling able to move more freely, full of energy and fit to take on the day.

Even when busy I can take time to make sure I eat things that are good for me and make me feel good and nourished afterwards.

I am committed to this more than ever now because this is a reflection of the Real Me, the one who is free of fear and limitation, the person I was born to be.

[Big cheer!]

Now, in this example we started off wanting to transform our health and well-being, but – three levels deep – ended up focusing on our sense of self-worth; and in transforming that, felt more in control, which in turn enabled the more surface-level transformation in our health and well-being to take place.

When we dig deeper, what we really want will always come down to one or more of our core beliefs. If there is resistance, it will also be at this level.

Part 2 and Part 3

Repeat the 'Three Levels Deep' exercise now for each 'one thing' that needs to change with regards to your DW/DW exercises on Career and Money, and Relationships and Intimacy. Record your answers in your journal on new pages, in the same way as you have done for Part 1 on Health and Well-being. Be sure to create updated summary statements for each.

Exercise 23: Your REAL Don't Want/Do Wants

Duration: 15–20 minutes
Journal Required: Yes
Buddy Required: Not necessary

Background

Whenever we are seeking to make change, it will be because we want to *feel* different in some way, and if we dig deep enough, it will always involve wanting to move from a negative core belief to a more positive core belief. As soon as we can acknowledge this, life gets a whole lot easier because you just have to work out which one it is and focus on that.

Instructions

Go back to your original DW/DW exercises in your journal, where you did one for each of the three categories of Health and Well-being, Career and Money, and Relationships and Intimacy.

Look at each pair of statements – 'Don't Wants' and 'Do Wants' – and in the middle column, which was previously blank, make a note of which core belief or beliefs are most relevant.

Take into account the information you uncovered from the 'Three Levels Deep' exercises, but ask yourself, 'Is this about my sense of "Enoughness"? Safeness? Control? Acceptance? Pleasure? En-lightenment?' If you are not sure, apply the 'Three Levels Deep' exercise to each idea, statement or 'wish' you are focusing on.

Be sure to do this because I want you to recognize how simple everything actually is.

- We think we want to change our health and well-being . . . but what we really want is to change one or more core beliefs.
- We think we want to change our career and money situation . . . but what we really want is to change one or more core beliefs.
- We think we want to change our relationship and intimacy situation . . . but what we really want to change is one or more core beliefs.

We think we need to change something on the outside to help us feel better on the inside. But, in fact, to get from where we are to where we want to be on the outside – *and stay there* – we must actually focus on the inside and bring about a transformation at the core belief level.

However we do so, and at whichever level of the U-Flow we are operating, we must let go of a layer of fear or limitation reflecting an old negative core belief and instead adopt or allow a new, more positive one to take its place. We must let go of a layer of the fearful you, who has been hypnotized and conditioned by life, and instead allow a greater connection to the Real You, one who is lighter and more free.

It is this more liberated you that will actually enable you to have different thoughts, experience different feelings and adopt different behaviours, which will ultimately help to create different outcomes in your life, more in alignment with what you really want.

However complicated life may seem on the surface, underneath it all comes down to a handful of ideas we hold about ourselves and about life, many of which were never even true in the first place.

Stepping Stone Beliefs

Earlier I said that I noticed people skipping a step in the DW/DW exercise. By that, I mean that instead of writing down opposites, they would write down two phrases that *were* 'Don't Wants' and 'Do Wants', but not opposites. For example:

DON'T WANT		DO WANT
Feel anxious		Be successful (?)

Anxious and successful are not opposites. When we do something like this, however much effort or persistence we apply, by jumping ahead and skipping a vital step we will only ever be wasting our time. The result is usually *wishful thinking* rather than *positive thinking*, and instead of crossing the drawbridge into the castle, we find the drawbridge is raised and we end up in the moat, feeling upset and sorry for ourselves.

In order to turn this from wishful thinking (which gives us something nice to think about but rarely achieves anything constructive) into positive thinking, which will inspire and motivate us to take positive action, there is a gap that must be filled.

There are a number of ways we can find out what needs to go in the gap. A simple method might be to ask a few questions:

- What do I need to think, feel or believe in order to be successful?
- What is the connection between feeling anxious and not being successful?
- What do we mean by 'successful' anyway, and why do we see that as opposite to being anxious?
- What would 'being successful' allow us to feel, that we currently do not?

An exploration of your answers or a discussion with an E.S.C.A.P.E. Buddy will usually reveal what is really going on.

We could also apply the 'Three Levels Deep' exercise to this:

	OLD	NEW
Current situation	Anxious	Willing to have a go, see what happens, go for it.
What's that like?	Frustrating, annoying because I hold myself back.	I can feel safer having a go, without fear of rejection.
Where does that leave you? What outcome?	Not doing things or achieving things I could, feel like a failure.	I may have failed but it doesn't make me a failure. I am enough whatever I do.

Now we find that the opposite of success (failure) is there, but three levels deep on the other side. And the opposite of anxious (safe having a go) is there, but two levels deep on the *other* side. But now we know what is really going on, we can plug that back into our DW/DW exercise and fill in the gap. These ideas act like stepping stones, helping us get from one side to the other, hence we can call them 'stepping stone beliefs'. Note the slight change of headings as we do so:

DON'T WANT	STEPPING STONE BELIEF	WHICH MEANS THAT
Feel anxious	I am **enough** whatever I do. I can feel **safe** having a go, without fear of **rejection**.	I can do the things required to be successful.

I'm sure you have noticed already, but the stepping stone beliefs will always be related to one or more of the core beliefs – in this example, 'Enoughness', Safeness and Acceptance.

Previously, if we had focused purely on being successful, the threat response would have kicked in subconsciously and most likely caused us to sabotage our efforts, avoid taking action or procrastinate. By focusing on the stepping stone beliefs instead, and increasing our sense of 'enoughness', safeness and acceptance, whatever happens, we can feel more free to give it a go and take the necessary actions to bring about the successful outcome we desire.

Exercise 24: Stepping Stone Beliefs

Duration: 15–20 minutes
Journal Required: Yes
Buddy Required: Can be helpful to spot anomalies that we cannot see ourselves

Background

Sometimes when we do the DW/DW exercise, our 'Do Wants' and 'Don't Wants' are not actually opposites. When this happens there is usually a gap that needs to be filled by what we can call a 'stepping stone belief'. Identifying where this happens and filling that gap is vital if we are to achieve a successful outcome. In such cases, it is the stepping stone belief that will actually allow us to create or achieve the thing we think we want!

Instructions

Look back over your DW/DW exercises and check for anywhere that the 'Don't Wants' and 'Do Wants' are not actually opposites. It may be helpful to have someone objective like your E.S.C.A.P.E. Buddy do this for you, because otherwise your threat response may create subtle resistance to facing up to the gap, accepting things at face value, wanting you to skip the exercise.

If you spot an anomaly, ask the following type of questions:

- What do I need to think, feel or believe in order to have/be [the 'Do Want']?
- What is the connection between these non-opposing 'Don't Wants' and 'Do Wants'?

- What do I mean by [the 'Do Want'] and why do I see that as opposite to [the 'Don't Want']?
- What would having/being [the 'Do Want'] allow me to feel that I currently do not?

For any that you identify, do a 'Three Levels Deep' exercise (see p. 234) to help identify what core belief you think you need to act as a stepping stone belief for you, in order to get to where you want, and then update your journal accordingly. If all of this sounds complicated, it is – and it isn't. All the time we are simply asking . . .

If you want to get from here . . . to *here* . . . and stay there . . . what is currently holding you back or stopping you, and what do you need to accept or believe instead that will finally allow you to achieve success?

All these exercises are geared to that end, but our critical faculty can jump in at any moment and activate the threat response, which is why we have to keep checking for, and digging into, every possibility of resistance.

There is just one more exercise we need to do on this for now. Earlier on we mentioned the idea of secondary gains causing conflicts, so let's just do an exercise to check for any of those now as well.

Exercise 25: Checking for Secondary Gains

Duration: 15–20 minutes
Journal Required: Yes
Buddy Required: Optional

Background

If you are still experiencing any resistance when you read through your 'Do Wants', it is important to check for secondary gains. A secondary gain is where, on the surface, our issue seems like a problem, but underneath it is actually serving a purpose and protecting us in a way we are fearful about letting go of, as in the weight loss example earlier, where feeling unattractive was helping to maintain safeness.

If any of your 'Do Wants' will take you away from a positive core belief and towards a negative one, you will feel resistance. To dissolve the resistance you must be able to resolve the conflict so that a move towards the 'Do Wants' will only increase positive core beliefs.

Instructions

Read through your DW/DW exercises in each of the three main areas of Health and Well-being, Career and Money, and Relationships and Intimacy, and check for any inner fear or resistance as you do.

Focus on your 'Do Wants' and ask yourself:

- Is there anything I am afraid will happen if I do this? If so, what?
- Is there anything I am afraid I will have to feel? If so, what?
- Is there anything I am afraid I am giving up? If so, what?

Again, this is really important because it is the little details like this that make a huge difference when attempting to create change.

Sometimes it will not be obvious that we have fears or reservations, but our body will always tell us if we are prepared to listen and take notice. The threat response will send subtle – or not so subtle – signals, such as tension, stress, a twitch, an ache, pain or sensation as we read through ideas that challenge our beliefs.

Do a 'Three Levels Deep' exercise (see p. 234) on any of the ideas that trigger this and identify if you perceive that moving towards the 'Do Wants' will involve the loss of a positive core belief, or the increase of a negative one.

Write the answers as a summary statement like this:

- I really want to [your 'Do Want'] but am afraid that if I do then I will [your fear/loss].

In the weight loss example we used earlier, it would be:

- I really want to lose weight but am afraid I will feel unsafe if I do.

Ask yourself:

- What do I need to feel, believe or accept to make it OK to move towards my 'Do Want'?

The answer will usually be the opposite of the old negative core belief – i.e. unsafe becomes safe, out of control becomes in control.

When you've got your answer, you need to write it down as a 'but actually' statement, and also change the 'old fear' part of the sentence into the past tense by using 'until now'.

- I really want to [your 'Do Want'] and until now have been afraid that if I do then I will [your fear/loss] but actually [new core belief about it].

For example:

- I really want to lose weight and until now have been afraid I will feel unsafe if I do but actually <u>it is safe for me to lose weight now, so I can.</u>

The underlined bit is all we really need to focus on and then our behaviours can follow – provided there is no internal resistance to the idea from anything we haven't covered yet.

Whenever I am doing this type of exercise, my ultimate aim is to help someone get from 'I couldn't . . .' to '. . . but now I can'.

- I couldn't lose weight . . . but now I can!
- I couldn't make my health a priority . . . but now I can!
- I couldn't perform well at work . . . but now I can!
- I couldn't allow myself to have a loving relationship . . . but now I can!

And so on.

We must be sure to do this thoroughly for each of the three main areas of Health and Well-being, Career and Money, Relationships and Intimacy, lest we fall prey to subconscious resistance. Remember, any time we are willing to face up to something, with persistence, on the other side of the fear is freedom.

Now, if all these 'Don't Wants' and 'Do Wants' seem a little wordy and overcomplicated, there is another way we can do this, which is often even quicker. Read on to find out about Life Metaphors and the Metaphormosis Technique, but you need to have grasped the DW/DW concept properly for it to work.

Life Metaphors

Sometimes it is useful to be able to take our problems outside of us, examine them objectively and then put them back in an improved, and ideally transformed, new way. A simple but effective way to do this is through the use of similes and metaphors. Grammatically, a simile is where we say we are 'like' something, whereas a metaphor says we 'are' that something. Both are OK, but the metaphor seems to be more impactful.

- In court, she was *like* a lioness = simile
- In court, she *was* a lioness = metaphor

- In the ring, he was *like* a raging bull = simile
- In the ring, he *was* a raging bull = metaphor

I have often used these 'life metaphors' to help clients make Identity Switches, especially where they have to change roles quite dramatically, such as in sports or business situations.

- As a father, I am a playful bear . . . as a premiership footballer, I am a deadly cheetah.

The formula is basically 'In one role, I am this, but in another role, I am *this!*' and you can apply it to any area or situation in life. With men, it is amazing how often James Bond is mentioned!

As an exercise, let's apply this to our three main areas we have been talking about because good imagery or a metaphor here can really help to cement our wordier exercises from earlier.

Exercise 26: Creating Your Life Metaphors

Duration: 5 minutes
Journal Required: Yes
Buddy Required: Not needed but may be helpful if you need an idea

Background

Having a metaphor for certain areas of life can help us draw on the characteristics of the metaphor we choose, embuing us with the qualities we aspire to.

Instructions

Part 1

1. For each of the three main areas of Health and Well-being, Career and Money, and Relationships and Intimacy, think of a person, animal, object or anything your imagination conjures up that will serve as a useful metaphor for how you want to be when the Real You is fully realized and activated in each of these areas.
2. For each one you choose, make a note of the qualities you aspire to that made you choose that metaphor or metaphors.

An example might be:

	METAPHOR	QUALITIES
Health and Well-being	I am a martial artist	Disciplined, agile, strong, powerful, calm, still

| Career and Money | I am an arrow | Focused, aiming for the target, unwavering, true |
| Relationships and Intimacy | I am an open book | Open to all, available to all, nothing to hide, a blank canvas |

Please do not skip this. By forcing yourself to do this, you are forcing your subconscious to face up to things and help bring about deeper and more lasting transformations for you.

Part 2

Repeat this any time you wish for any area of life where you play different roles, especially if you need to 'step up' and perform in some way. It is also OK to draw on the qualities of more than one person or object, and combine them together.

Make a note of any such roles and associated metaphors in your journal.

Life metaphors can be incredibly powerful tools for reinforcing positive ideas – but what if our life metaphor, when we think of it, is negative?

That's where the next exercise comes in beautifully. By combining the 'Life Metaphors' exercise with the 'Three Levels Deep' exercise, we can often get an incredible metamorphosis, often very quickly. Hence the name of this next method – the Metaphormosis Technique.

Exercise 27: The Metaphormosis Technique

Duration: 10–15 minutes
Journal Required: Yes
Buddy Required: Can be really helpful, provided they ask questions and do not give too many suggestions

Background

Some people like to use a lot of metaphors and these can be incredibly effective tools for transformation in themselves. In the Metaphormosis Technique we do a 'Three Levels Deep' style exercise but using *only metaphors*.

For example, here's what came out when I did this on one of my courses recently.

ME: Describe the current situation.

STUDENT: When I fight with my daughter and we are at loggerheads, it feels like a runaway train, about to fall off the tracks of harmony.

ME: What's that like?

STUDENT: Fast-moving, everything going too quickly.

ME: What's the result or outcome?

STUDENT: A big crash!

ME: OK, instead of being in a big crash, what do you want instead?

STUDENT: I'd rather be in a sailing boat.

ME: What's that like?

STUDENT: Slower, more in control, gentle breeze, calm waters.

ME: So how does the situation begin to feel now?

STUDENT: More like smooth sailing, teamwork, together.

We then created a summary idea to take away and focus on.

ME: Any time you sense you are at loggerheads with your daughter, instead of allowing it to become like a runaway train, moving too quickly and destined to crash . . . take a deep breath and, as you breathe out, think of the idea of a sailing boat, moving slowly, more in control in the gentle breeze and calm waters, so that you can work together, as a team, and things can be more like plain sailing.

Instructions

1. For each of the three main areas of Health and Well-being,
   Career and Money, Relationships and Intimacy, complete a
   'Three Levels Deep' exercise but ONLY using metaphors.

   You can use other words, including feelings and emotions, while
   you are working through it, but only put the metaphor in the 'Three
   Levels Deep' grid. For many people this is not easy, but I have found
   it to be always worth the effort of persisting.

   It is usually easier to let a simile arise naturally, while describing something. For example, one of my students was saying that
   she was afraid of getting fitter and healthier because she knew that
   would give her more energy, and she felt scared about that. 'My
   energy is something separate from me, like a coiled spring,' she said,
   'and I've been a bit like a sad sloth,' so we put that in our first box,
   even though technically it is a simile.

	OLD	NEW
(1) Current situation metaphor	Like a sad sloth, with my energy separate, like a coiled spring.	
(2) *What's that like?* metaphor		
(3) *Where does that leave you?* metaphor		

2. Next ask the questions at each level, going down levels 1, 2 and
   3 on the left-hand side, creating a metaphor or simile for each
   one.
3. When you have completed the left-hand side, ask yourself,
   'Instead of [old Level 3 outcome imagery] what would be a
   better image, a better metaphor?' Write the answer in the new
   Level 3 box.

4. Now, with that new Level 3 metaphor, ask, 'What's that like?' and create an image for that, writing it in the new Level 2 box, as we move back up.
5. Finally, think about the impact of that and allow a new metaphor to form of the new situation.
6. Create a summary statement that basically says: 'If ever you start to feel [your old current situation metaphor], instead you can now think of [your new current situation metaphor].'

Here is the example from above now completed. If you can do this for *any* area of life where you currently have a challenge or difficulty, as well as the three main areas we have been focusing on, it will open up options for you and create new perspectives. **The end result will also be an image or metaphor that more closely reflects the Real You, free of fear and limitation, now able to be more of the person you were born to be.**

	OLD	NEW
(1) Current situation metaphor	Like a sad sloth, with my energy separate, like a coiled spring	A hippopotamus and a butterfly! (see explanation below)
(2) *What's that like?* metaphor	(Too dangerous to let out) It could explode at any moment and destroy me	Like a rainbow, inspirational, with creative energy
(3) *Where does that leave you?* metaphor	(Destroyed . . .) Like a squashed frog!	(Instead of a squashed frog . . .) I'd rather be a triumphant angel, with one of those big trumpet things

So my student went from a sad sloth, with energy separate like a dangerously coiled spring, to the sturdiness of a hippopotamus combined with the transience of a butterfly, with the energy being more inspirational, 'more me' she said, which means it is OK for her to have more energy now by getting fitter and healthier.

At first these can seem weird . . . but you will only understand the full transformational impact if you do this yourself! And one more thing to recognize: core beliefs were involved again here, moving from energy being unsafe and out of control to feeling safe and in control. Very often, to get from the old to the new, we must ask ourselves, *'What do I need to think, feel, believe or accept in order to take on board the new idea and, in particular, which core belief do I need to accept or focus on?'*

The exercises until now have largely been very solution-focused, dealing with thoughts, beliefs and ideas in the present, without particularly needing to dig into the past. However, we will find it difficult to create lasting success and change if we are still holding on to highly charged memories and experiences which our mind is using as a reference point for how to be and what to expect. Having conducted in excess of 17,000 one-to-one sessions, I have seen that accessing a root cause idea, using regression to evoke memories, is one of the fastest and most effective ways to bring about deep and lasting transformations, so let's look a little more closely at this now and discover how you can apply it to your own situation.

Same Feeling – Different Story

If you think back to the U-Flow, what we were trying to do was figure out the best place to help ourselves break these loops and patterns of thinking. One of the initial things I also look for with clients is examples of what we can call 'Same Feeling – Different Story'.

By this I mean that, even though the situation, the people, the events, the conversations and actions that make up a particular story or event in our lives may be entirely different, the feelings or emotions we are left with are the same and may give clues as to where the issues are really coming from.

In a client session, I would most likely help the client relax and go inward, then use regression to follow the feelings back to their causes, going through a Don't Want/Do Want-type approach, down there, at that level, but I do not want to encourage you to do that without professional guidance. Although we can get dramatic results doing that, the process itself can get quite dramatic at times. However, there is still a lot you can do yourself and in a moment we will do an exercise on this. But, first, a quick case study to help illustrate.

CASE STUDY: *Samantha Gets a Pay Rise*

When twenty-six-year-old Samantha asked me for help she was working in the bespoke jewellery business. An expert in her field, she often travelled the world sourcing unique gems to create stunningly beautiful diamond rings, hand-crafted jewelled necklaces or priceless-looking bracelets for clients of the prestigious company she worked for.

'I love diamonds,' she told me with a sparkle in her own eyes and I could see she meant it wholeheartedly. 'And I love my job and I love the company I work for,' she went on. 'But I am being paid way below the level I should be for what I do and I'm terrified to ask for a raise. I did ask once but he only gave me 1 per cent and it felt like an insult and showed huge lack of respect.'

The more I questioned her, the more I realized this was way more than an everyday case of someone feeling nervous about asking for a raise; this was more than just nerves. As she described the situation to me, she began displaying signs of high anxiety, panic and tearfulness even just talking about it.

When I asked her to close her eyes, relax and go inward, and to follow the feelings, we first went back to a scene where she was asking to borrow some money from her grandpa for the deposit on a flat.

She used exactly the same words to describe the scene – terrified, out of control, powerless, can't speak – as she did when speaking about asking for a pay rise, and so we had a good example of a different story, but the same feeling.

I dug deeper still and we found her back aged six or seven, having to ask her dad for some money for something, and feeling exactly the same way – intense anxiety and wanting to avoid his gaze, as if she had done something terribly wrong. Again, same feeling, different story.

And following that feeling down further still, we found a scene where she was very little and felt she was being told off for *who she was*, rather than something she had done, causing her to feel as if there was something intrinsically wrong with her (i.e. not enough) and this had begun to feel like a recurring theme as a child. Something about the way her dad had responded that day when she asked for money linked the two together, and so asking for money and her being intrinsically wrong as a person had become linked together. Twenty-something years later, she was feeling exactly the same way when thinking about asking her boss for a pay rise and subconsciously she had given it the same meaning as asking for money from her dad or grandpa.

As I took her through this, the fear and shame of that little self came pouring out. With the release of the emotion, we could help that young childhood version of herself see the situation for what it really was, rather than the false opinion she had formed of it, and with that she began to relax and feel better.

As she realized there was nothing actually wrong with her and it was OK to ask for things sometimes, including money when it was needed, the idea of asking for a pay rise that she knew she well and truly deserved suddenly seemed much more acceptable, as she was now able to give it a different meaning.

The following week she arrived with an even bigger smile than usual, reporting that first thing the morning after the previous week's class she had asked for a meeting with her boss. She had presented her case calmly and confidently, and he had agreed to the full amount of the pay rise, without objection, effectively doubling her salary!

Very often, when we no longer subconsciously expect others to behave in a certain way towards us or around us, it is as if others subconsciously pick up on that and adjust their behaviour accordingly. We then no longer seek out or draw towards us experiences that recreate the old feeling. Instead, we break the loop and begin to seek out or draw towards us new experiences that resonate with the new feelings – in Samantha's case, self-worth, confidence and value.

I have used the same process that I used with Samantha many thousands of times to rid people of addictions, traumas, self-sabotage, anxiety, panic, abuse and a whole host of other symptoms and problems, including many physical ailments, by accessing the underlying beliefs and emotions that are being triggered to create the surface-level symptoms – sometimes in just one or two sessions, sometimes over a number of weeks or months, depending on the particular case.

We don't need to access the emotional memories with every issue, but it can be a very fast way to bring about deep change, especially when there is evidence of repeating patterns. It is probably *the kindest, quickest and most effective way of clearing past traumas* that I know, especially when combined with other exercises, and can save years of conventional therapy and treatments.

For now, let's go through something to help you if you feel there is an unresolved issue from your past that is still affecting you.

Exercise 28: Following the Feelings

Duration: 30–60 minutes
Journal Required: Yes
Buddy Required: Can be helpful

Background

If we are finding it difficult to make changes at the surface level, it may be that we are still holding on to meaningful memories or traumas. Sometimes there may be just one or sometimes it can be an accumulation of events. If we can identify anywhere that we are having the same feelings now as we had in the past – same feeling, different story – it can give us an idea of where to look in order to finally be able to let go and move on.

Instructions

What we are eventually looking for are situations where the story, people and events may be different in themselves, but the feelings and emotions we experience are the same or similar.

Start off, however, by thinking about that 'one thing' that needs to change in each of your three main areas (Health, Career, Relationships), and on a new page in your journal write down the most reactive, throwaway comment that comes to mind for each. For example, these would be a great start:

- 'I can't lose weight.'
- 'I have an idiot boss.'
- 'I will never feel satisfied in my relationship.'

Sometimes the inner self-talk or throwaway comments we make when we encounter these situations are actual word-for-word statements of our invisible beliefs. But more often than not the initial throwaway comment or reaction is a description of the surface-level symptom.

As we now know, we can work at this level with the DW/DW or we can use the 'Three Levels Deep' exercise or the Metaphormosis Technique to probe a little deeper to get the best results possible, but either way it is usually beneficial to expand on this initial statement before attempting to dig deeper into it.

Once we have our initial comment or outburst we need to write down a description of what we mean by it, in as much detail as we can muster. This is more of an outpouring or rant rather than the more structured 'Three Levels Deep' type exercises, although we are achieving a similar aim.

To get the real benefit, we need to convey as much feeling and emotive content as possible. Feelings and emotions are the manifestations of our beliefs – **follow the feelings and we will find our beliefs**.

And, by the way, just *thinking* about doing this is not the same as actually expressing it, either verbally or in writing. When working with clients, I nearly always ask them to speak ideas out loud, often repeating phrases numerous times because it greatly enhances the effectiveness of the process. So if it is useful, for the purposes of this exercise, you can imagine you are writing it to me or you can record it using a voice note on your phone or other device and just imagine you are telling someone.

If you are working with a Buddy, you can use them, provided it is someone you trust and they are willing to listen without prejudice, as described earlier. There is something about the sharing of our inner thoughts and demons with another that is more powerful and more cathartic than doing so alone.

And by the way, if you feel any resistance to this process – fantastic! That resistance is actually a flag waving, saying, 'Dig here!' So make sure you begin this exercise by expressing the resistance as well. For example, 'I really cannot see the point in doing this exercise but . . .'

Remember, also, you are doing this for you, not me. (And maybe the species as a whole, but no pressure – evolution usually takes a few million years so no rush!)

Take time to get into this properly. If it helps, take a few deep breaths and close your eyes as we have done before. Think about what it has been like to be you. Think about the thoughts and feelings you experience on the inside as a result of what is occurring on the outside and express it in as much detail as possible.

'I can't lose weight' becomes:

I have no willpower. Every day I start off with the best intention but by the end of the day, when I finally sit down, I just want to snack and drink and have a treat. It's like I don't care and say to myself I'll start tomorrow instead. I think it's the only time I have just for me. The rest of the day I am taking care of everyone and everything, but in the evening I finally get home, have some time to myself and I just want to feel good. Sometimes it's the only time I get to think as well and, as I don't always like what comes to mind, I eat to take my mind off it. When I look in the mirror I just feel like an ugly, unattractive failure. Losing weight is so hard!

'My boss is an idiot' becomes:

I get so frustrated at work. It seems no matter how much work I do or how hard I try, it is never enough, and my boss just never listens. I have a lot of knowledge and experience to offer, but my boss seems to take all the credit and all the money for what I do. It is unfair. It's like I am never fully appreciated and beating my head against a wall. It makes me so angry and, like, what's the point? And if I ask for something he will never give it to me. I feel helpless.

'I will never feel satisfied in my relationship' becomes:

I love my husband, but he is never going to satisfy me in the way I want. He is emotionless and never shows he cares – I wish he would show some affection or make me feel loved and that he does care. I just want to escape and it makes me think of being with someone else. In the past I have spent hours daydreaming and fantasizing about it and even getting close to someone, and I am worried that I may eventually do something that would ruin the family and upset my children. I feel stuck, trapped. He is so like my father and I don't think he is capable of changing.

Now, once we have finished this initial expressing, we need to go back through what we have written and underline or circle any emotive phrases or elements that are likely to create emotion. For example, 'My boss is an idiot':

I get so <u>frustrated</u> at work. It seems no matter how much work I do or how hard I try, it is <u>never enough</u>, and my boss just <u>never listens</u>. I have a lot of knowledge and experience to offer, but my boss seems to take all the credit and all the money for what I do. It is <u>unfair</u>. It's like I am <u>never fully appreciated</u> and <u>beating my head against a wall</u>. It makes me so <u>angry</u> and, like, <u>what's the point</u>? And <u>if I ask for something he will never give it to me</u>. I feel <u>helpless</u>.

Let's take all these emotive words out:

- frustrated
- never enough
- never listens
- unfair
- never fully appreciated
- beating my head against a wall
- angry
- what's the point
- if I ask for something he will never give it to me
- helpless

When you have your list of emotive words or phrases, just focus on the feelings, without the story, and feel around for any familiarity.

- Do these feelings seem familiar to you?
- Do you recognize them?

- Can you feel, sense, picture or imagine other times where you have felt the same or similar?
- In your recent years?
- As a young adult?
- As a teenager?
- As a child?

Don't wrack your brain to remember something – that won't work. And besides, it's actually not the memory we are interested in – it is the emotionally charged ideas, the beliefs with emotions wrapped around, that we are after.

Make this an effortless process. Just think about what it feels like to be you – and follow the feelings to wherever they take you. You may find it easier to say this out loud first, rather than writing, to keep the flow going.

Here is our other example, 'I can't lose weight':

I have no willpower. Every day I start off with the best intention but by the end of the day, when I finally sit down, <u>I just want to snack and drink and have a treat</u>. It's like <u>I don't care</u> and say to myself I'll start tomorrow instead. I think it's the <u>only time I have just for me</u>. The rest of the day I am <u>taking care of everyone and everything</u>, but in the evening I finally get some <u>time to myself</u> and I just <u>want to feel good</u>. Sometimes it's the only time I get to think as well and, as <u>I don't always like what comes to mind</u>, I <u>eat to take my mind off it</u>. When I look in the mirror I just feel like an <u>ugly, unattractive failure</u>. <u>Losing weight is so hard</u>.

- I just want to . . . have a treat
- I don't care
- only time I have just for me
- taking care of everyone and everything
- time to myself
- want to feel good
- I don't always like what comes to mind
- eat to take my mind off it

- ugly, unattractive failure
- losing weight is so hard

And finally, 'I will never feel satisfied in my relationship':

I love my husband, but he is never going to satisfy me in the way I want. He is emotionless and never shows he cares – I wish he would show some affection or make me feel loved and that he does care. I just want to escape and it makes me think of being with someone else. In the past I have spent hours daydreaming and fantasizing about it and even getting close to someone, and I am worried that I may eventually do something that would ruin the family and upset my children. I feel stuck, trapped. He is so like my father.

- I love
- never going to satisfy me
- emotionless
- never shows he cares
- wish he would show some affection
- make me feel loved
- and that he does care
- being with someone else
- daydreaming and fantasizing
- feel stuck, trapped
- like my father

In a session with a client, these are the words and phrases I am looking out for and will dig into, whether with DW/DW, 'Three Levels Deep' or 'Following the Feelings'. For the purposes of this exercise, follow these feelings to where they take you and, in your journal, note any memories that come to mind.

If your mind links back to them when following the feeling, it is a pretty good bet that your mind – your inner librarian – is using these memories as a reference for what to do and how to be, and is providing supportive evidence as to why you need to think, feel and behave the way you do.

Accessing these can sometimes be very painful at first, but remember, if we can identify the feelings and release them rather than reacting to them, we can finally be free. The more you can stay with the feelings and find a way to express the raw emotive content, the more likely you are to have a cathartic response, where you feel lighter and freer as a result.

NOTE: If it feels too much or too scary, you should seek professional help so you can do this in a safe way, where you feel guided and supported. Please refer to the 'Next Step' section at the back of the book (p. 319) for more guidance on this.

What we are looking for in this initial outpouring, and any associated memories that come to mind, is evidence of the threat response, core beliefs or what I call 'statements of belief'.

A statement of belief is something we say as if it is a fact, although actually it is usually just a strongly held belief.

- 'I'm a failure.'
- 'Getting fit is impossible.'
- 'I will never find love.'

Anytime I hear one of these, I usually just ask, 'In what way?' and use something like the 'Three Levels Deep' approach to elicit what is going on behind it. If we only try to deal with it at the surface level, we will probably encounter anger – resistance – fear.

'I'm a failure.'
'No, you're not.'
'Yes, I am!!'

'Getting fit is impossible.'
'No, it isn't, you just have to –'
'That's all right for you to say!'

'I will never find love.'
'Of course you will.'
'Really? Then why haven't I so far?!'

The threat response will kick in as the statement is challenged directly. But if you dig deeper you will usually get to the raw, emotive content of the idea or memories and be able to initiate a more productive resolution.

If we can identify which of the core beliefs are being acted out, we can also refer to the relevant 'Increasing Your Sense of . . .' exercise to help remedy that.

Once we have a deeper understanding of what is really going on, our original statement of belief can usually soften and we can test if a new idea can begin to form by adding 'Until now' and 'but actually' once again. For example: 'Until now I have believed that [old statement of belief] . . . but actually [new insight] . . .'

For example:

- Until now I have believed that my boss is an idiot but actually I am just frustrated because I undervalue myself and I am not getting a chance to 'prove my worth' properly. If I value my own worth more, my boss will reflect that back to me, or I will find a new job somewhere else instead.
- Until now I have believed that getting fit is impossible but actually it is easy under the right conditions. I have been afraid to stop comfort eating and drinking so much because of the scared or lonely feeling I feel, but if I can deal with that, I can change my eating behaviours and start exercising, and getting fit will be much easier.
- Until now I have believed that I can never get what I really need from my relationship but actually when I can accept myself more, I can relax and accept my partner more and discover there is much more love there than I realized, and we can become closer than I had previously believed was possible.

In each case there will have been a fear – a negative core belief – behind the statement of belief, and the statement itself was really a form of the threat response, thinking it was protecting us from feeling pain, while actually preventing us from feeling worth, value and love.

For many of us doing this exercise, a new belief will open up . . . and that new belief, that new idea, however alien it may seem at first, is something we can use, latch on to, reinforce, repeat, focus on, so that it eventually becomes more acceptable and then more normal.

There are many, many exercises we can do to work with any difficult memories that come up, and I use a variety of these with clients, usually while they are relaxed, eyes closed and focused inward. One of the simplest and most effective processes you can do yourself is a collection of short exercises which, when run together, form what I call a 'Releasing the Past' exercise.

Exercise 29: Releasing the Past

Duration: 20–30 minutes
Journal Required: Yes
Buddy Required: Optional

Background

If we store emotionally charged memories, they will usually be fuelling our beliefs, affecting how we think, feel and behave, but those same memories can often keep an aspect of us stuck, locked, imprisoned in time, destined to feel the same way again and again.

When we can release any suppressed or repressed emotion around such memories, we can set this previously imprisoned aspect of ourself free. The emotional driving force behind any issues that have arisen can then reduce or dissolve away, allowing any old surface-level symptoms to dissolve with them and new, more desirable outcomes can then take their place.

I first came across the concept of the 'inner child' in my early hypno days when I met author Penny Parks and read her book *Rescuing the Inner Child*, which is excellent for anyone who has suffered any childhood abuse or trauma. Over the years, I have adapted and developed my own approach, and this is the process I take people through as we *follow the feelings* deeper. It usually consists of four parts:

1. Establishing a connection
2. Expressing the unexpressed
3. Giving back the feelings
4. Powering the inner voice

Part 1 – Establishing a Connection

When you find a memory of a younger you – and younger could mean any time from a few days ago, right the way until early childhood – the first step is to form a connection to that 'you'.

1. This time take a few deep breaths in and out through your *mouth*, making you more emotionally open and possibly even feeling a little vulnerable.
2. Make the out-breath longer than the in-breath, so that it feels like a very gentle sigh of relief.
3. Close your eyes as you breathe out and go within, allowing the muscles of your body to relax as you do.
4. Maintain the breathing for several more of these sigh-of-relief-type breaths.
5. Pay attention to any thoughts that come up for you, but as you breathe out, imagine blowing them away and refocusing your attention on to your breath.
6. Tell your body to *relax*. (Sometimes it is easier to tell our bodies to relax than it is to tell ourselves to relax.)
7. After a few more normal breaths, let your mind focus deeper within yourself and feel around for a place deep within, away from the normal world, beyond the thoughts and fears and limitations of your life. Feel around for that sense of peace that is always there and you can always return to.

When you feel ready, think about that memory or scene that has been troubling you. Now imagine you can go back in time. If you wish, you can take someone you trust with you. Imagine you are walking into that scene and walking up to younger you. You do not need to picture or imagine this vividly, just a sense of it will do. Imagine walking up to that younger you, looking into their eyes and saying:

I know what it feels like to be you. I know what you are thinking, I know what you are feeling, I know what you are afraid of right now, and I know exactly what it feels like to be you right now, because I AM you. We are just different perspectives of the same person and I have come to help you. I have come to help you, and be with you, so that you do not need to feel alone with this any more. We can sort this out together.

Very often this will create a wave of emotion, often a mixture of sadness and comfort. If it feels appropriate, imagine giving that younger you a hug.

Part 2: Expressing the Unexpressed

The aim of this part is to help the younger you express any feelings or emotions that have been held in or 'unexpressed' until now.

It is important to understand that we are not looking for the polite version, the kind you might tell someone you meet who asks you about a certain area of life. And we are not talking about intellectual analysis, the kind we might have in a therapeutic discussion.

What we need is the real, gritty, uncensored, raw, emotive content of the experience, in whichever words or language come out. (This is where clients have often laughed afterwards, telling me, 'I didn't know I was allowed to say those kind of words in therapy!')

What we want is a purging, so that any idea that took root in the subconscious is uprooted and set free. Imagine you and that younger you turning towards whoever or whatever is causing the distress to the younger you and telling them exactly how you feel. Say to them: 'When you [whatever it is they do], you make me feel [whatever it is they make you feel],' and let it all flood out.

I know many spiritual teachings say practise forgiveness, and of course there is a place for that, but I have always found it virtually impossible to even contemplate forgiveness while we still hold hurt and resentment. Deal with the honest feelings – the hurts, the pains, the anger, the betrayals – face them, bring them to the surface, express them, release them in a safe way like this, and then they will no longer be with you – or to a lesser degree at least.

Also, I know technically nobody can be *made* to feel anything, but in reality, when horrible stuff happens in real life, it certainly feels as if someone or something is making us feel that way – and when we access it, it can feel that way all over again, so let's respond in the natural way in order to be free of it.

If you prefer, you can do this by writing it down, as in a letter, but *you do not need to send it*. Just purge the feelings and emotions, expressed towards the original source of them.

If you feel hatred, it's OK, express the hatred.

'I hate you for making me feel this way,' might be appropriate for some.

For others, 'I love you but I hate the way you make me feel,' might sit easier.

If you feel scared to do this, begin the sentence with: 'I feel scared to do this, but . . .' and then continue.

If you feel guilty doing this, begin with: 'I feel guilty saying this, but . . .' and then continue.

There are no rules other than . . . DO NOT ASK A QUESTION!

Do not say, 'Why did you do this? Why did this happen to me?' because that is usually counterproductive, and I'll explain why shortly. Just make it about expressing or verbalizing what you feel. Express the unexpressed until there is nothing left to say.

Part 3: Giving Back the Feelings

Once you have made a connection to that inner, younger you, and stood with them as they express whatever they have been carrying inside, imagine now gathering up all these feelings you have been speaking about and, as you breathe out, *sending them back to whoever or whatever caused them*, so that they now have to feel them instead.

Do this several times, or for as long as it takes; long, slow, deep breaths, sending the feelings back to where they came from. A teacher? A parent? A sibling? A 'friend'? A partner? An ex? A stranger?

What you want is for the person to feel whatever they made you feel . . . not to punish but for you to find peace.

If it is a stranger or someone you are not that close to, imagine saying to them, 'These are your feelings, you gave them to me, but I do not want them any more. Take them back and go and deal with them!' or words to that effect.

If it is someone closer to you, you can amend it to say, 'I don't want you to feel this for ever, I just want you to feel it so that you understand, and never do it again, then we can both be free,' or something like that.

This can often be very emotional, but when it hits the spot, you will find it a very cathartic experience.

I usually check in to see how the client is feeling as they do this, and this is where we often get the 'lighter, freer, taller' sort of comments.

Once you have done this and feel a sense of relief or release, we need to connect that back to where we started and do what I call 'Powering the Inner Voice'.

Part 4 – Powering the Inner Voice

Once you have connected to that inner you, helped express anything that was previously unexpressed and given the feelings back to where they came from, you are usually in a place where you can begin to feel different. This is where I am now looking for an 'I can' statement.

'Now that you have done this, and you feel lighter and freer, what does it mean about that issue we were talking about earlier?'

'It means that now I can [be myself/feel more confident/go for the job/eat more sensibly/feel safe with a partner, etc.]'

I want you to power up your inner voice with a new mantra that actually feels real and means something to you, indicating that something has now changed for you.

'Before I couldn't . . . but now I can!'

Any time we release our past in this way, we are undoing some conditioning, dehypnotizing ourselves from how we thought life had to be and opening up to new ways of how it can be from now on.

This is most definitely not always easy, but in the same way that some of the most beautiful beaches are the hardest to find, some of the deepest, most profound releases we experience can be found by having the courage to veer off the well-trodden path and being brave enough to face what we find there. Because on the other side of that is a level of calmness and peace we have often not felt for a very long time.

Exercise 30: Forgiveness

Duration: 5 minutes
Journal Required: No
Buddy Required: No

Background

To find peace, ultimately we must feel forgiveness, but not in the usual meaning of the word. The typical interpretation of forgiveness is to say, 'You have done something wrong, but I will be gracious enough to let you off any ill feeling. *I will wrap you in a ball of forgiving light,*' and so on.

Lovely though this is in theory, very often that ill-feeling is subconsciously still there, which is why I check for any unexpressed resentment when dealing with past memories so that we can get a truer, deeper forgiveness.

However, I have come to understand there is a deeper level still, and true forgiveness means being able to view an experience as if it *never even happened.* Not 'overlooked' or 'I'll let you off this time'. For true peace and forgiveness we must be able to think and feel as if the incident or experience that has been causing us upset never even took place. Not repressed or suppressed either – it must be viewed as if it never happened, which takes forgiveness to another level, one that most of us find difficult to accept at first.

This may seem strange, but very often we are holding on to grievances because holding on to them actually gives us something – usually something relating to a core belief – and we are afraid that if we truly forgive, we will lose that thing we think we are gaining. But, in fact, the opposite occurs, and when we can truly forgive in this way, we find peace.

This doesn't mean we just allow people to keep doing things to us; it doesn't mean we condone certain behaviours. It *does* mean, ideally, we can move on in such a way that the grievance has no meaning and we do not seek it out any more, thus breaking the cycle. There are many ways to dehypnotize ourselves and find new ways of being, and this is another.

Instructions

1. Find a quiet place where you will not be disturbed. You can do this sitting with eyes closed, or walking around if you prefer, as long as you're somewhere you can be alone with your thoughts.
2. Set a timer on your phone or other device for five minutes, and for those five minutes let your mind feel around for anyone or anything causing you anger.
3. Try to avoid getting caught up in the drama of the thoughts, just ask yourself, '*What would it feel like if I could let this person go on their way, as if it had never even happened?*' and pay attention to what that makes you feel. Anger? Fear? Loss of power? Losing face?

4. Ask yourself again, *'What would it feel like if I could let this person go on their way, as if it had never even happened . . . and instead just feel peace?'*
5. See if you can hold on to the 'peace' feeling for more than a moment . . . each second you hold on to it, you are helping to break the cycle of whatever it is you feel you are needing to forgive.

This forgiveness feeling should not only come from your head and your heart, but you should feel it in your guts too, which is where many of our resentments are held.

If you feel tension anywhere doing this, see if you can let go another level deeper. You will need to let go of any notion of being right, or of judgement, or of seeking revenge, or of wanting an apology or anything like that. Any of these, or similar, will indicate an intellectual attempt at forgiveness, while maintaining a subconscious resentment.

If you have a genuine desire to forgive, but it is still too raw, that is fine. Try, 'I want to forgive you, and will do when the time is right,' or words to that effect. Remember, we are not saying that what they did was OK! We are saying that we want to let it go from our psyche so completely, it can feel as if it never even happened, so that we are completely free of it. Not blotting it out but free because we no longer attach any meaning to it (think back to our very first exercise on 'Awareness of Meaning').

If it is just too difficult, that is fine too. Acknowledge why it is difficult and use whichever of the previous exercises seems appropriate to dig into it.

The one thing we do *not* want to do is fake forgiveness because that just goes into our subconscious and causes more problems. If we still have an issue, it means one or more of our core beliefs is being challenged. That is OK, just sit with the feeling, be mindful of it, then do a DW/DW around that and see what comes up.

Ultimately, we just want to be at peace with the situation, and that is the aim.

Exercise 31: *The U-Flow Summary*

Duration: Hard to tell!
Journal Required: Yes
Buddy Required: Optional

Background

Finally, we are back here with the U-Flow! In the previous sections and exercises I have been giving you the various pieces of the jigsaw puzzle to do this yourself, so let's put that together now and see how this can go to work on easing or solving some of the issues in your life.

Let's use our three main category ideas of Health and Well-being, Career and Money, and Relationships and Intimacy for one final time.

Using the blank template on p. 276 as a guide, or drawing one out in your journal, complete a U-Flow for the 'one thing' that *needs* to change in each of the three main areas.

You will already have many of the answers you need from previous exercises, but you may need to repeat some in order to get a more focused result.

Be sure to do this exercise in an externally expressive way. Don't just do it in your head because otherwise it will just stay in your head. Make the effort to write down the answers in your journal. If there is an E.S.C.A.P.E. Buddy you can trust, work together as instructed – taking turns to answer the questions out loud – but paying attention any time either of you leave a sentence unfinished or a word interrupted. Be sure to finish the word or sentence – it will help bring the invisible to the surface and make it visible and more accessible.

Instructions

1. Beginning with Health and Well-being, think about that 'one thing' that needs to change.

2. In the top left, write out your surface-level symptoms that you wish to change. What is it you want to *stop* or *reduce*, your 'Don't Want'?

3. From your DW/DW exercise on this, write in your new, opposite 'Do Want' in the desired outcome box.

4. Move to the next level down and write down your old 'Don't Want' thoughts, feelings, emotions, actions and behaviours you are aware of that have been contributing to those surface-level symptoms. You may have uncovered these in your 'Three Levels Deep' exercises.

5. On the other side of the page, write down your new, positive answers from the 'Three Levels Deep' exercises.

6. Moving down a level further, on the left side write down what you must have been *believing* in order to be thinking, feeling and behaving in that way. Any statements of belief might go here.

7. On the other side, write down your new statements of belief, that do allow for the change. This might be a summary of your 'but actually' statement from the 'Statement of Beliefs' exercise.

8. Drop down another level and write down any memories, life experiences or internal references that seem to have been supporting any statements of belief.

9. On the other side, write down your 'I can' statements from the 'Releasing the Past' exercise.

10. At the bottom, write down any old core beliefs associated with the old surface-level symptoms. You will find these in 'Your Real Don't Want/Do Wants' exercise and 'Secondary Gains' exercise, if relevant.

11. Write down which core beliefs you will be seeking to increase by changing this area of your life.

12. Write down your old Identity Statement associated with the old way of being, from your 'How to Reveal Your Invisible Identities' exercise.

13. On the other side, write down your new Identity Statement.

14. Once you have a completed U-Flow, *read it from the bottom up on the right-hand side*. Often, starting with the positive core

beliefs will lead to variations or new ideas further up that will actually be more meaningful and more transformational for you.

15. Take a break if you wish, then repeat for the other two areas of Career and Money, and Relationships and Intimacy.

16. Give yourself a pat on the back.

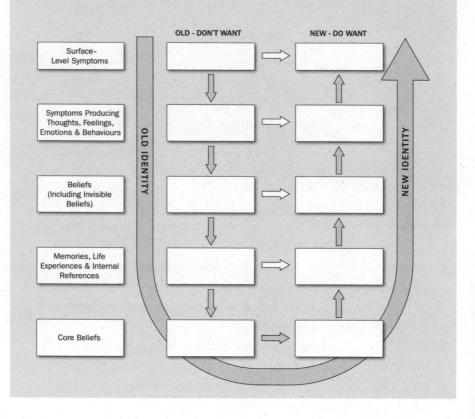

Rules of Success

In any endeavour we wish to accomplish, there are rules of success for achieving it. If we follow the rules, we will likely achieve success. If we don't, we won't. In sports motivation it is sometimes called 'process not result', i.e. don't focus on the end result (winning), focus on the process to get there (eat well, train hard, positive psychology, rest and recovery) and everything else will take care of itself.

If there is something you wish to change about yourself or your life, there will be 'Rules of Success' for achieving it. If you look at your U-Flow now, on the right-hand side it should give you the rules to follow and focus on for achieving success in that area, or making progress that way at the very least.

If you have a big enough 'Why' and feel an appropriate level of commitment, you should feel inspired to think, feel and behave differently in some way. A way that will create more of the right conditions for achieving that which you wish to achieve. If you still feel resistance in any area, that's fine, remember your 'Why' and dig deeper into the resistance, as we have done before, asking yourself, 'What am I thinking, what am I feeling, what am I believing? What do I need to think/feel/believe instead?'

When all levels of the U-Flow finally line up, you will be more likely to create the right conditions that will lead to a more positive, successful outcome.

All Hypnosis is Really Self-Hypnosis

There are many books on hypnotherapy and hypnosis, but I didn't want to write one of those. I wanted to write a book on transforming lives because that is what really interests me and natural hypnosis is merely a tool we can use to aid that.

In reality, all hypnosis is self-hypnosis and all of us are already experts. Every time we focus on an idea, unchallenged, and allow that idea to take root in our subconscious, that is hypnosis, whether we pay someone to say things to us, listen to a recording or say it to ourselves, amidst one of the many thousands of thoughts we have each day.

Our conscious mind focuses on the idea, and it is the conscious focus on it that allows it to take root. To repeat, we are not knocked unconscious, but we may lose or lower our critical faculty for a while if the conditions are right.

Unfortunately, fear, shock and trauma provide the perfect conditions for hypnosis, along with constant repetition, which is why we can become hypnotized by life and conditioned to respond, usually as a reflection of our upbringing or significant events.

While many would have you believe otherwise, there is no mystical state, just a very naturally occurring shift of focus from one reality to another, which some find easier to do than others.

If you wish to carry out a formal self-hypnosis session, to reinforce the ideas from the U-Flow, you can do so using any of the methods already described for helping you to relax, slow down your breathing and go inward.

Some people will say we have to do little tricks to get past the critical faculty, but really, the critical faculty is trying to protect you, so why trick it? Understand it, educate it, and it will gladly step aside and become your ally.

Self-hypnotic Questions

I have heard it said from many sources and in many ways that the quality of our life will be determined by the quality of what we focus on, and that certainly rings true from my experience. But I have also heard it said that the quality of our life will be determined by the quality of the *questions* we ask ourself because whenever we ask ourself a question, something interesting happens – our mind will go looking for an answer!

The way the question is phrased will also determine the answer we go looking for – and ultimately determine what we end up focusing on.

For example, if we make a mistake through lack of concentration or any other reason, we could easily say to ourselves, 'Ah – how could I be so stupid?', and our mind will go searching for an answer for us, looking for reasons as to why we are so stupid, doing its best to search our life experiences and beliefs for reasons to explain why we are so stupid.

'Well, you're an idiot so of course you are stupid. You never listen, you never concentrate, you never have done, and now you've got to work even harder because you messed up in the first place. You're such an idiot.'

Another example could be, 'Why is it that nobody likes me?'

'Well, you're very unlovable, so who is going to like you? Think of all the times when you've felt unlovable or unliked and it's obvious. There's something wrong with you, you're not normal. You're never going to be liked so what's the point in trying?'

We may not always be aware of the answer, but we will probably feel it, or our reaction to it at least – which will most likely be a threat response, creating a surface-level symptom. It may be momentary or it may remain, niggling away at us for some time as we continue berating ourselves. Interestingly, as I mistyped that last sentence the spellchecker corrected the word 'berating' to 'betraying'. And that is what we are doing every time we berate ourselves in that way – we are betraying ourselves.

The conscious or subconscious self-talk that follows one of these self-critical questions will always be a reflection of some of our beliefs – often the invisible ones that operate and exist in plain sight but we just cannot see – so such questions are actually yet another way we can begin to make the invisible, visible.

But these kinds of questions will always set our minds looking for evidence or ideas to justify or fulfil the *context* of the question, and will usually leave us feeling whatever the negative focus of the question was – 'stupid' and 'unloved' in our two examples above – and the various spin-offs from that.

By asking questions in this negative way we are actually rehypnotizing ourselves or reconditioning ourselves to believe the negative idea even more strongly. Because it feels real and valid in that moment, the ideas barge straight past the critical faculty – the gatekeeper – and into the club, where they can dance the night away. And we only feel the effect in our feelings and emotions that follow, rather than the instant fight or flight reaction we would feel if the gatekeeper didn't accept them.

Such questions are like an indirect suggestion. 'How could I be so stupid?' is essentially saying 'I am stupid'. 'Why is it that nobody likes me?' is saying, 'Nobody likes me,' and we accept the idea without challenge.

But what if we could use the same phenomenon *for* us, instead of against us? What if we could interrupt that old, automatic process and replace it with a different question? One with a more positive, more desirable context? What if we could ask a question that sent our mind off looking for an answer, but the answer was something we wanted, rather than didn't want? What would our mind do then?

- How can I become someone who makes health and happiness their priority?
- How can I create a more satisfying and rewarding career?
- How can I bring more love into my current relationship?

And what if we attached a meaning to it as well? A 'so that'?

- How can I allow myself to concentrate better . . . so that I can get more things right first time?

- How can I appreciate that people do like me . . . so that I can feel more relaxed in social situations?
- How can I become more accepting of others . . . so that I can become more accepting of myself?

The general formula is:

How can I think/feel [something more positive] so that I can [have a more desirable outcome]?

There may be a little resistance to begin with but, with persistence, the focus switches to the new, more desirable idea and the subconscious goes looking to support it and act upon it.

It is important, however, that *we do not go looking for the answer to the question!* That is not the aim, initially. The aim is to get the idea and the *feeling* of the idea accepted, focused on, *without being challenged.* Then we get natural hypnosis occurring.

Remember, whatever we focus on or give energy to will make us think, feel and behave in such a way that we tend to bring more of that into our life. Phrasing what we *want* as a question, in this way, helps to lower our critical faculty even further and begins to plant the seed of a new idea or new belief in our conscious and subconscious mind.

We do not need to do this all the time, but for many of us, a positively phrased self-hypnotic question will work way better than a more conventional positive-thinking-type statement or affirmation because the critical faculty has a reduced reaction to it.

Think of the effect of being able to focus on the words in these questions:

- What do I need to do to *get this done on time?*
- How can I *make the team this week?*
- What are three ways I have been a *kind and likeable person* this week?
- How can I *see this differently?*

Again, we are not necessarily looking for an answer – it is the *feeling of asking the question* we are interested in right now.

For many people, a few repetitions of asking a self-hypnotic question will be quite transformational, especially at easing or managing symptoms. For others, it will plant the seed of a much deeper transformation.

In some people, however, it will trigger deeper resistance, and when that happens, we just have to dig deeper still. The question will usually initiate a useful flow of information at the very least.

Remember the principle from the DW/DW exercise, as well, where the 'Do Want' always needs to be positively phrased. For example, rather than 'How can I not feel anxious?' (which emphasizes the word 'anxious'), much better would be 'How can I stay *calm and relaxed*?', which gives emphasis to the words 'calm and relaxed'.

Can we use this in everyday life too? Absolutely. My other grandfather, who was not a prisoner of war, told me how he used this exact process to solve a major production-line problem in the British motor industry when he was a young toolmaker, back in the 1930s. Production of cars was being severely held up because a special tool was needed but no one could figure out how to make it. Everyone was baffled and pressure was mounting for my grandfather's department to come up with a solution.

'I couldn't think of the answer,' he explained, 'but what I could do was clearly define the problem, and with that, I could then more clearly define what we needed, even though I didn't yet know how to bring it about. After clarifying both the problem and what we needed, I went to sleep, holding the problem in my mind, asking myself the question, "How can we make the tool to provide the solution we need so that production can continue?"'

What happened next is fascinating and a topic worthy of a book in itself. He awoke in the middle of the night with the solution absolutely clear in his mind. He sat up in bed, made a rough sketch on a piece of paper so as not to forget it, and then went back to sleep. In the morning he made a more detailed drawing and then presented his solution on arrival at work that morning. It worked. The tool was made, production continued, and my grandfather gained an instant promotion to head of the department. I must give him credit for introducing me to the concept of self-hypnotic questions – though the name came from me!

Exercise 32: Self-hypnotic Questions

Duration: 5–10 minutes
Journal Required: Yes
Buddy Required: Not really

Background

By turning a positively phrased statement into a question, it can help us focus on the positive idea without triggering resistance, while also encouraging our subconscious mind to go seeking for answers.

Instructions

1. Look back at your Don't Want/Do Want lists now and see if you can convert any of the 'Do Want' statements into self-hypnotic questions by adding a question at the beginning, such as 'How can I . . .'. For example, 'How can I make my health even more of a priority now?' (The 'even more' is an idea I picked up from a Tony Robbins recording, when describing a similar process.)
2. Make a note of these self-hypnotic questions in your journal and read them like a prescription two or three times a day until they stick in your mind and you can recall them at will.
3. Any time you come across any challenge in your daily life, think about what outcome you want and practise asking about it as a self-hypnotic question.

Exercise 33: Take Five in Five

Duration: 1–2 minutes
Journal Required: No
Buddy Required: No

Background

This is an exercise I may introduce to clients to help them cope or manage symptoms, while we are working on change at a deeper level. But it can actually be extremely effective at creating long-term benefit in itself, especially if carried out persistently. And if used in conjunction with the 'Awareness of Meaning' exercise or the DW/DW process, or as a tag-on to one of the deeper sessions, it can really help nudge people forward in their transformation process. Its beauty is in its simplicity.

Instructions

1. ANY time you catch yourself thinking one of your old, negative, 'Don't Want' thoughts or ideas – or any new ones that come to mind – within five seconds of becoming aware, take a deep breath and, on the first exhale, become aware of any meaning you are attaching to the event or idea that is creating tension or anxiety.
2. See if you can identify which of the core beliefs is being activated as you do. Lack of 'Enoughness'? Safety? Control? Acceptance? Pleasure? En-lightenment?
3. Continue with another four deep breaths, and on each exhale now, go through the 'I don't want to think/feel this, I want to think/feel *this*' process, using whatever comes to mind or a statement from your earlier exercises. You could even use a self-hypnotic question.

NOTE: You do not have to take five breaths in five seconds, you just have to *start the process* within five seconds of noticing the original negative thought, and take five breaths overall.

Is this time-consuming? Yes. Is it repetitive? Yes. Is it boring? Yes, at first. Is it worth it? You will only know that if you do it. Sometimes, you may not have the time for five breaths – that's OK – but be sure to do at least one breath within five seconds of becoming aware of the original thought.

Do this and you are setting yourself free, moment by moment, thought by thought, breaking the old patterns and meanings and introducing new ones, every single day, until one day, you discover you do not need to do it any more. Because the Real You does not need to do any of this.

PART THREE

The Mind and Body

Our Psychology Affects Our Biology

So far we have talked about personal, emotional and behavioural problems, and how our thoughts, beliefs and the threat response impact these, creating a whole array of surface-level symptoms. But one area that has always fascinated me is the influence our psychology can have on our biology.

One of the first books I ever read on this was *The Psychobiology of Mind–Body Healing*, by Dr Ernest Rossi, where I learned about neuro-peptides, messenger molecules and details of the long-term effect of stress on the body. A few years earlier, when I was twenty-one, my father had died of a heart attack, to be followed two months later by my mother, of a brain tumour, both aged only forty-seven.

It was a terrible shock and catapulted me and my life on to a completely new trajectory. If we include the effect of being adopted, I had now lost my second set of parents, and I believe it was this that set me on the rather self-destructive path that followed for a number of years until I 'crashed' and found myself responding to the 'Find out about hypnosis' voice I heard that day I mentioned in the Introduction.

Studying mind–body medicine, I couldn't believe that this information was not more widely available or taught at school. Our thoughts can play a part in the development of illness? Or, conversely, contribute towards health? Or even switch off pain? Surely not. And yet the evidence seemed to suggest this was so.

Back in 1841, for example, a Scottish-born physician named James Braid became intrigued by a strange phenomenon he witnessed at a demonstration where the performer, one Charles Lafontaine, was claiming the ability to make his volunteer subjects impervious to pain. Braid was sceptical, and rightly so. The demonstration was actually a recreation of the methods introduced nearly seventy years previously by the German doctor Franz Anton Mesmer. Mesmer charmed the courts of Europe with his ability to heal, at first by passing magnets around the subject's body, and then eventually dispensing with the magnets, just by using a dramatic waving and passing of his hands, attempting to realign the misaligned 'animal magnetism' within the patients' bodies – an idea that actually bears some resemblance to Chinese medicine theories.

During this process, the subjects would seem to go into a trance-like, sleep-like state, where they appeared to be responsive to the instructions of the operator – and it is from this Mesmer state that we get the word 'mesmerized'.

Although Mesmer's theories and explanations did not sit comfortably with Braid, he did become fascinated by the trance-like appearance of some of the volunteers in the demonstration he witnessed. Trying to find a scientific explanation for the strange phenomenon, he began carrying out private experiments of his own, practising on his wife, friends, servants and patients.

One of the bizarre procedures he developed for recreating the state he had witnessed involved strapping a cork to the patient's forehead and asking them to focus on it by rolling their eyes up. It would often take a few minutes of this before the patient was 'ready' and instructed to close their eyes, but once in the required state, the responsive patient was more positively affected by the things he said, including maintaining raised arms or legs, though he wrote that 'responsiveness varied considerably from person to person'.

The eye-closure element made it appear that the subjects were asleep and so he used the Greek god of sleep – Hypnos – as a name for this state, hence the term 'hypnosis' was born.

He eventually realized that the state he was creating had nothing to do with sleep and more to do with helping the patient focus their mind around *one idea* – monoideism – to the exclusion of all others. When they did this, he could more readily help them elicit the desired response on their body.

Although monoideism was Braid's preferred description for the phenomenon, the press at the time were having none of it and latched on to the original one of hypnosis, saying his patients had been hypnotized, which was subsequently widely adopted around Europe. With images of their arms outstretched and eyes closed or rolled up, perhaps you can now understand where the old movie portrayals originate!

Braid later amended his methods and thankfully did away with both the cork and the outstretched arms, but wrote detailed accounts of being able to help and heal a number of conditions through this use of focus and imagination. These included alleviating pain, treating rheumatoid conditions, easing skin complaints and even curvature of the spine. I myself have been able to assist with something similar, to a certain degree, with a volunteer on my very first training course. The gentleman described the sensation as if his spine was 'unwinding like a corkscrew' and he walked out of the room a very different person to the one who had hobbled in with a walking stick. Although the effect seemed quite miraculous, by having the client go inward and visualize what he wanted, I was actually just teaching the body to unwind itself. I'll go through a few methods you can use yourself shortly.

The problem is that individual results like this are not always replicable, which makes them difficult to quantify and difficult to accept medically, but there are those seeking to correct this. Take a look at the work of Wim Hof, for example, holder of twenty-six world records related to mind–body endurance and phenomena. Wim was able to resist the effect of an endotoxin injected into his bloodstream that should have created an inflammation response, but his body showed no symptoms. And to prove it wasn't a fluke, he trained twelve others to do the same. Using Hof's methods, volunteers were able to dramatically increase their level of epinephrine, which is believed to be the suppressor of the inflammatory agent of the endotoxins. Controlling the immune system in this way is something the medical world has deemed impossible, yet on numerous occasions, and under strict scientific research conditions, he has shown we can consciously, deliberately influence our immune system when we are willing to learn how.

Wim is known as the Ice Man owing to his association with ice baths and cold showers, along with climbing Mount Everest wearing only shorts and sandals! I can barely do him justice here, but what he teaches to all his students and followers is the ability to adapt: 'By learning how to adapt to the cold, we can train ourselves to adapt to the stresses of life. Our body is capable of so much more than we realize.' With twenty-six world records to his name, it is very difficult to argue or disagree. Combined with breathing techniques and mindset, Wim has developed very simple protocols that we can all employ, which push the boundaries of what we thought was possible with respect to physical and mental health. He is a true pioneer and I highly recommend his book, *The Wim Hof Method*.

The Placebo or Belief Response

Prior to the Second World War many doctors and physicians had already been quietly prescribing sugar pills or similar in order to placate certain patients, whom they considered did not actually warrant the treatment they were seeking. But when some of these patients actually began to recover after taking these pills, it seemed a whole new phenomenon had been discovered, though largely ignored at first.

Then, in a US field hospital during the latter part of the Second World War, anaesthetist Dr Henry Beecher and his staff were overwhelmed by the number of casualties being brought to them. Morphine was the standard injection to relieve pain and it was effective, creating almost instant relief (I, too, have enjoyed its benefits myself when recovering from a painful procedure). But when Beecher's supplies ran out one day and a nurse spontaneously decided to administer a saline injection instead to the wounded soldier lying on the operating table before them, Beecher was surprised to discover that the salt solution had exactly the same effect as the morphine – creating near instant pain relief in the traumatized soldier, despite there being no active pain-relieving ingredient. They repeated this process many times whenever morphine supplies were low or ran out.

Returning home after the war, this effect intrigued Beecher and he began to investigate how much of a patient's response to a drug was from the drug itself and how much was down to the *idea* of taking a drug. Around this time, others such as Harry Gold at Cornell University were also taking an interest and beginning studies.

It seems incredible now, but until Beecher published his report in 1955, the pharmaceutical industry had never had to test their drugs against a dummy version to find out how much of the benefit was down to the drug and how much was down to the *idea* of having received the drug.

In many cases, when patients *believed* they were getting a valid medication, they and their bodies seemed to respond exactly as if they had received the real medication, even though there was no active ingredient present. Nowadays, we know this as the Placebo Response or Placebo Effect, from the Latin for 'I please', but it should really be called the Belief Response or Belief Effect.

There are already numerous books on this topic but they largely stop at the observation of what is happening, without being able to give instruction on how to create it ourselves. This is again worthy of a book in itself but in a moment I will give you some techniques you can experiment with – provided you have already been checked out medically so that you do not suppress symptoms of a more serious underlying condition that does need medical attention.

However, there are some very important subtleties we need to note, and it is a lack of understanding of these, I feel, that has caused confusion among the numerous studies that have been carried out to ascertain the authenticity of the Belief Effect.

Long before Beecher's discovery, in the late 1880s, French pharmacist Émile Coué began treating patients, free of charge, using a form of autosuggestion, where he did away with the need for any kind of formal hypnotic state entirely.

Coué's approach was very simple – he obtained absolute focus of attention and then asked the patient to repeatedly concentrate on one idea and one idea alone (sound familiar?) by repeating a certain phrase out loud, twenty times in the morning and twenty times in the evening. The phrase was: *'Tous les jours à tous points de vue je vais de mieux en mieux.'*

Translated to English, it is: 'Every day, in every way, I am getting better and better.'

It was probably one of the earliest forms of a modern-day health affirmation, and reports estimate Coué treated somewhere between twenty to forty thousand people in this way, initially individually, later in groups.

> We possess within us a force of incalculable power, which if we direct it
> in a conscious and wise manner, gives us the mastery of ourselves and
> allows us not only to escape from physical and mental ills, but also to live
> in relative happiness

states Coué, but qualifies it with,

When the imagination and willpower are in conflict, are antagonistic, it is always the imagination which wins, without any exception.

This is the bit that most people miss and, I feel, is why placebo trials are often misleading.

If our conscious will desires one thing but the imagination – that inner, often invisible, subconscious voice or imagery – holds a different idea, we will once again be running up that down escalator, and the down escalator – the subconscious imagination – will eventually win.

Coué instructed that we have to focus on that ONE idea and ONE idea alone – we cannot just say the words while secretly thinking something else – the will and the imagination must be in alignment. These are the conditions for natural hypnosis to occur, when the ideas we focus on meet no internal resistance from the critical faculty or gatekeeper of the mind.

He also pointed out that there were two types of autosuggestion, as he called it. One is a deliberate, formal version, as in the 'Every day in every way I am getting better and better' exercise, and the other is the more subtle, often subconscious way that we repeat ideas to ourselves without even realizing – our inner self-talk or inner imagery.

In terms we have been using so far, the first one involves us having to consciously and deliberately find some way to reduce or bypass that critical faculty, the gatekeeper of the mind. The latter way slips past unnoticed! But, again, both are using the same process we have been referring to throughout this book.

Coué would also use these techniques to encourage patients to expect more positive results from any medication they were taking – supporting the medical treatment, rather than replacing it – and if more health professionals could understand the benefit of this nowadays, we might have less fear and less resistance around the notion of adopting some of these ideas.

Focusing on an idea twenty times without becoming distracted is actually quite difficult, so Coué suggested we take a small piece of rope or cord and tie twenty knots in it. We then move our hands along each knot, each time we say the phrase. I did try this but got bored after a few days and then lost the cord!

Fortunately, once we grasp the principles, we can employ these ideas to great effect in much more relaxed ways. I think the ritual is often important to begin with but can then be dispensed with once we have internalized a shortcut for it. However, this process can also seem to work in very mysterious ways . . .

A BBC *Horizon* documentary entitled 'Placebo' told the story of a medical secretary from the US who had been suffering with severe IBS – irritable bowel syndrome – and was invited to take part in a trial to test the effect of placebos – inert sugar pills – on the IBS, *even while knowing it was a placebo.*

Amazingly, within three days the woman's symptoms had completely disappeared and remained so while she was on the trial. The pain, bloating, cramps and other effects had all vanished. Tragically, when the trial ended and the supply of placebos ran out, her symptoms returned to where they were before!

The documentary ends with a shot of her sadly trying to seek out more placebos. All this poor lady needs is someone to give her a different ritual, one that she can believe in, to create the same effect.

This documentary also explained how the appearance of the placebo can have different effects, stating that capsules tend to work better than round pills, with red capsules working best for pain, while blue capsules work best for anxiety.

Other studies have even shown the placebo effect to be at work in surgery as well, with people recovering from sham arthritic knee surgery just as well as those who had the real operation, going on to play sports and regain physical movement where previously they were unable or in great pain. The same has been shown to be true for some back surgery too.

A more extreme example of this is the case of 'The Likeable Mr Wright', reported by Dr Bruno Klopfer in 1957, which I first read about in Ernest Rossi's book mentioned earlier. The patient, Mr Wright, was suffering with cancer of the lymph nodes and in the very last stages of his disease, with little hope of recovery. Bedridden with large tumours, fluid on the lungs and difficulty breathing, Wright was ineligible for standard treatments of the time owing to his anaemia, and so was literally wasting away, waiting to die. But he had a strong spirit about him and, on overhearing talk of a new wonder drug called Krebiozen, pleaded with Klopfer to be included in the trials. Incredibly, three days after receiving the injections, Klopfer reports that Wright was up and about, walking, talking, laughing and joking, his tumours having 'melted like snowballs'. Ten days after the Krebiozen, he was discharged and declared cancer free, able to pick up his life.

Two months later, however, reports hit the news about rumours of the new wonder drug not being as effective as first thought and the effect on Wright was dramatic. His tumours returned and he was readmitted to hospital shortly afterwards, once again under the care of Dr Klopfer.

Klopfer was intrigued by what had happened before and so came up with a plan. He told Wright that a new, more potent version of the drug had just been released and that he had a sample to try, if Wright was willing.

Of course, he was. Klopfer created a ritual around the procedure, as if it were real, injecting him with saltwater – the same saline solution used in the field hospital by Henry Beecher and staff in place of morphine – and waited to see what would happen.

Again, the results were incredible – Wright made a full recovery and was discharged from hospital.

The great tragedy is that, sometime after this, reports confirmed Krebiozen as being completely useless, Wright's faith was lost, his cancer returned and he died.

This is an extreme example and one that is difficult to replicate – but there are many, many cases of people recovering from so-called incurable illnesses, which the medical world typically label as 'spontaneous remission', inferring that the illness suddenly disappeared all by itself. Can we really just 'wish' disease and illness away, if we really believe hard enough? That would be nice but closer investigation reveals there is much more going on.

Your thoughts – your words – your imagination – can have a profound effect on your body and, if the conditions are right, that effect can be extremely dramatic. In a moment I will give you a simple experiment you can try, adapting the principles of James Braid, Émile Coué and the

Belief Response to any area of physical discomfort you may be experiencing right now. But first, I want you to appreciate how simple this can be by looking at the case study of one of my students who decided to practise some pain relief techniques on his daughter.

CASE STUDY: *Natural Pain Relief*

When Kerry was thirty-three she developed pain in her lower back that grew steadily worse over the next three years. Despite numerous tests, medical professionals were unable to ascertain the cause and so diagnosed chronic pain disorder.

Her doctors prescribed painkillers starting with co-codamol, then as the pain got worse they upped them to tramadol, then to Zomorph. Finally, about five years after the pain initially started, she was put on Oramorph as well, an oral form of morphine that she could use as a booster during the day if needed.

Kerry's father, Richard Phillips, had booked on to my practitioner course and explained how the doctors now wanted Kerry to reduce the Oramorph and Zomorph and try to manage the pain herself. Kerry was concerned and asked her dad if he could help, using hypnosis.

Richard explains, 'I went to visit my daughter and just described how the treatment works, regarding imagination. I then asked her some questions about the pain she wanted some assistance with.'

Kerry's current medication regime was 40mg Zomorph in the morning and 40mg in the evening, plus the Oramorph as and when required for additional pain relief, plus some antidepressants to help her cope with her feelings.

On the morning Richard turned up to visit his daughter, Kerry hadn't yet taken any pain medication in order to see how well her dad's treatment would work.

Richard helped Kerry to relax and go into that inwardly focused state, and then read her a script that gets the client to imagine a healing lake that they can visit and bathe in. As they immerse themselves in the lake, it gently takes away the pain and discomfort. It also reminds them that they can use their imagination to recreate this relief at any time to reinforce this.

Kerry's initial report immediately after the session was that the pain had disappeared, leaving just a slight aching, which was a vast improvement from prior to the session. Around half an hour later, she felt tired and drifted into a deep sleep for about an hour or so. This is also quite a common occurrence after a deep session, though people can often feel the complete opposite.

On waking from her sleep, Kerry reported that she was still feeling the same – no discomfort but a slight ache – and reported the same again seven hours later.

The next day, which was a Monday, she said she knew something was there but there was still no pain, which she described as feeling 'unusual'. It was the same for Tuesday and most of Wednesday – no pain, no discomfort and no medication!

On Wednesday evening she reported that although she knew her back pain was there, she still couldn't feel it; however, her lower legs and ankles were starting to feel discomfort, which hadn't been an issue before. Finally, that evening, she took 20mg of Zomorph – her first medication for nearly four days, since Richard had carried out the session with her.

In the days that followed the pain settled down and she was able to manage with 20mg of Zomorph in the morning and the same in the evening – but still no oral needed. So after an initial period of no morphine for four days, since the evening of the fourth day she had taken less than half of her original medication. Kerry still knows there is something there from the original area but still can't feel any *pain*.

The net result was that Kerry was able to be morphine-free for nearly four days after her dad read some words to her from a few bits of paper he had been given!

All hypnosis is really self-hypnosis, of course, so it was Kerry focusing on the ideas that actually created the result. Sometimes it really can be that simple.

Exercise 34: Creating the Belief Response

Duration: 15–20 minutes
Journal Required: Yes
Buddy Required: Not essential but can be helpful

IMPORTANT! Before carrying out this exercise, *please* make sure you have had a full medical diagnosis to ensure you do not mask any underlying issues that may need medical attention.

Background

When focused in the right way, our thoughts have a far greater impact on our bodies than most people realize. This exercise* is similar to what I do with clients to help them ease a chronic ache, pain or area of physical discomfort, so please only apply it to something like that at the moment. Treat it as an experiment, to see what happens. As you will discover, it is an adaptation of the Don't Want/Do Want exercise . . . but do not be fooled by the simplicity of it.

Instructions

NB: You will need a glass of water to do this exercise.

1. Think of an area of your body in which there may be some discomfort in some way. That is actually a suggestion already – we are changing the words ache/pain/hurt to 'discomfort' because the focus of that word is *comfort* (your mind will have a tendency to filter out the *dis*).

* Adapted from a method called Noesitherapy, pioneered by Spanish surgeon Dr Angel Escudero, who trained patients to create natural analgesia for surgery without anaesthetic, introduced to me by Dominic Beirne.

2. Focus on that area of discomfort and, if safe to do so, close your eyes, let your mind go inside your body and imagine that discomfort from an internal perspective. Imagine what it looks like or feels like. This does not need to be medically accurate at all – just use your imagination. See if you can get a few words that describe the sensation of it, for example:

> hot
> red
> raw
> sharp
> sore
> jagged

Or see if you can let your mind represent it in some way that means something to you:

> stuck
> twisted
> rigid
> knotted
> tight
> broken
> weak
> squashed
> trapped

What we are seeking to find is a way for your mind to represent the condition in a way that is meaningful to *you*.

- The pain in my shoulder is hot, red, sharp, like a dagger is sticking in.
- My stomach feels sore, bloated, painful, like it is heavy and full of something spiky and scratchy.
- My knee is stuck, rigid, locked, and filled with black tar.

Do this for yourself before proceeding. Take a moment to really get a feel and sense of what your inner experience of this condition is. Make sure you get at least three words to describe it and write them down in your journal. These are all of your 'Don't Wants'.

3. Now for each of these, you need to write down an opposite list, which will form your 'Do Wants', describing how you would like it to feel or how you imagine it looking instead, for example:

hot	=>	cool
red	=>	pale blue
raw	=>	healed
sharp	=>	smooth
sore	=>	soothed
jagged	=>	even
stuck	=>	free
twisted	=>	straight
rigid	=>	flexible
knotted	=>	unravelled
tight	=>	loose
broken	=>	fixed
weak	=>	strong
squashed	=>	released
trapped	=>	free

Your words may be similar to or completely different to my examples – go with the words that feel best to you.

NOTE: As an interim exercise . . . Read all the *negative* words from above in one continuous list and imagine them applied to your body, noticing any effect as you do. Many people will feel a negative impact from simply reading those words and thinking about their body. Now read the opposite, more *positive* list, and imagine those applied to your body, noticing any effect while you do.

Notice any difference? If you do, great, it shows you have the immediate potential for impacting your body in a positive way. If you didn't notice any difference, no worry. You may have been a little too analytical about the process or it may just not be relevant to you at the moment, which is even better!

But a high percentage of us will feel some difference simply from reading these two different lists. Can you imagine the long-term effect of that, whether for the negative or the positive?

OK, back to the main exercise.

4. We want to focus on the description of your condition and switch that to positives by stating what you *want* it to be, as far as possible replacing each and every negative with an equivalent, more desirable positive. Be sure to find an opposite for each descriptive word.

DON'T WANT OLD CONDITION	DO WANT NEW CONDITION
The pain in my shoulder is hot, red, sharp, like something is sticking in.	I want my shoulder to feel cool, pale blue, soft and free, like it is healed and normal.
My stomach feels sore, bloated, painful, like it is heavy and full of something spiky and scratchy.	I want my stomach to feel relaxed, comfortable, light, soft and smooth inside.
My knee is stuck, rigid, locked, and filled with black, like tar.	I want my knee to feel loose, flexible and free, filled with a beautiful yellow light, like honey.

5. Take a sip of the water and swill it around your mouth but do not swallow yet. As you do so, concentrate on the NEW condition you want to create, saying it to yourself as far as you can with a mouthful of water; as you do so, imagine you are infusing that effect into the mouthful of water, so that the water now embodies the idea of the condition you wish to create. For example, 'cool, pale blue, soft, free, healed and normal'.

6. Swallow the water and imagine the water is carrying the new positive condition down through your body, spreading 'cool, pale blue, soft, free, healed and normal' through your body and to the desired area. Really focus on this as you do so – ONE idea, remember?

7. Repeat steps 5 and 6 two more times, so three times in all. Then just get on with your day.
8. Do this twice a day, morning and evening, for about five days and see what happens.

Will it relieve your aches and pains? I don't know. Will it ease your condition? I don't know. What I do know is that some people reading this will have no benefit, some will have a partial benefit and some people will have a HUGE benefit.

There are many ways to implement the Belief Response and this is one of the simplest versions of the exercise I can explain in the space available here. With more time and more detail we can go deeper, and embed further, refining and fine-tuning, seeking out the approach that works best for each of us.

In a one-to-one session with a client, I would typically take up to forty minutes or so to really understand the specifics of how they experienced their condition and help them develop a bespoke procedure to help relieve their condition through psychological means.

But while these Belief Response exercises can be extremely effective at easing some symptoms for many people, I would not tend to use them myself for dealing with major illness. For providing psychological support for assisting more conventional treatments, I might wish to dig a little deeper. On occasion, we may even initiate a conversation between the client and the area of the body needing help – it is quite amazing what clients reveal when you ask them to give their physical ailment a voice! Sometimes we just have to go beyond the illness.

Beyond the Illness

Back in early 1985, when I was nineteen, I returned home from a week away with a friend to discover that my then forty-five-year-old mother could no longer read. She could identify and say the letters – R-E-D – but could no longer put them together to make a word. It was funny – at first. Then the headaches started. A week later she was rushed to hospital and I still remember the day my dad came home and told us she had been diagnosed with a cancerous brain tumour and given six weeks to live.

The first thing I did was to go and buy some cigarettes. I didn't even smoke but thought that was what people did when something shocking happened! It was the first and only pack I have ever bought but I always remember that when helping people stop smoking.

At the time, this cancer diagnosis *was* a shock – but looking back with what I know now, it shouldn't have been. All the signs were there that she was experiencing more and more stress, and feeling more and more unable to cope, experiencing feelings of desperation, isolation and depression, until eventually her body had said 'enough'. She died two years after her diagnosis.

Am I claiming that all cancerous brain tumours are down to stress? I have no evidence to support that but what I witnessed fits a pattern I have since become aware of, which is that in cases of major illness or disease, there are often a series of major life stresses occurring, starting around twelve to eighteen months prior to the eventual outbreak of symptoms.

The more we understand about the effect of our psychology on our biology, the more it makes sense that many diseases and illnesses do not just spontaneously happen, but that there is a pathway leading to them and the symptoms we eventually present to our doctor or medical practitioner are actually only one part of a much longer story.

There is a whole new area of medical research called epigenetics, which investigates how factors occurring outside of our cells can determine how the genes are activated or deactivated within our cells. These factors include toxins from the environment, and our nutrition, as well as the stress chemicals created by our psychology. Our environment, our diet, our emotions and even our willpower can have an impact on our genes and how they are activated or deactivated!

For anyone willing to look, there are countless documented cases of spontaneous remission, whereby someone's supposedly untreatable medical condition or illness spontaneously disappears or goes into remission, often baffling the medical specialists. The implication is that this happens suddenly, overnight, with no apparent explanation or cause – yet the deeper we are prepared to look into these cases, the more we discover that there is nothing random or spontaneous at all. There is a clearly defined shift that occurs in the patients' attitude and lifestyle, which impacts down to the cellular and even genetic level, thereby bringing about the biological changes required to ease or eliminate the previous symptoms. The same process in reverse is probably what caused the development of the condition in the first place. Dr Jeffrey Rediger's book *Cured* covers this in great detail, as do the writings of cancer surgeon Dr Bernie Siegel and back pain specialist Dr Sarno, to name a few.

Back in 2006 I was invited to take part in research into a cure for tinnitus, the ringing, whistling, buzzing, whooshing sound in the head that affects up to 10 per cent of the population. I'd had some previous success with this and there were a few testimonials on my website, which is how I became drawn in. I spent a great deal of time with many of the world's experts on this topic and even had an annual conference based around one of the ideas I put forward. But it was the words of a top surgeon from New Zealand that really struck home for me.

Sat in a conference room of a hotel in Valencia, at the inaugural meeting of what would become the Tinnitus Research Initiative, the surgeon picked up a pen and started to draw on a napkin for me. He drew a sketch of the brain with a shaded area for the amygdala – the emotional centre of the brain, the one connected with the threat response.

'It seems to me,' he explained, 'that whatever initially caused the tinnitus in the first place, as soon as it moves into the amygdala it forms a loop, which then sustains it, even if the original cause has long since disappeared.' And then, looking me in the eye: 'As a surgeon, I cannot operate on that area . . .'

'But I can!' I thought – that is how I had already managed to help some tinnitus sufferers and what I have continued to do.

To be clear, whenever people ask me for help with this, I say, 'I cannot cure your tinnitus, but I can help you create the right conditions so that it settles down, reduces or at the very least appears to reduce and drift into the background by itself.'

And all I do is take them through the E.S.C.A.P.E. Method, as already described. I help them access any underlying stress or emotions, even if they have nothing to do with the tinnitus directly, so that their inner stress levels calm down and reduce. And once we have done that, I use more conscious focusing to help them switch off the threat response, which often sustains the condition, and to focus away from the sound. It is not uncommon for someone to walk in with their tinnitus at 9 or 10 on a scale of 1–10, and walk out two or three sessions later with it down to a 3, a 2 or less.

There is currently no pill or potion on the planet that can do this; if there were it would be hailed as a miracle cure. But all we are doing is going beyond the illness or disease, treating it as any other surface-level symptom, and seeing what may be going on in the background.

Another of my graduates, Sara Loiperdinger, had a great experience recently, sending me the following text message after a session:

> Hi Andrew, I wanted to tell you that I gave my friend a session for pain relief. We did regression and some other great stuff, and released the anxiety, feelings and pain that had been there for over twenty years. He laughed, and cried, and said for the first time ever the pain has gone, and he knows it won't come back.

When I pressed for more details, Sara explained that her friend had experienced a traumatic incident as a child that had left him feeling he had done something wrong, and the headache pain in his temple had been there ever since and, in a way, was trying to protect him from thinking about the event or feeling those emotions.

As he released all the suppressed and repressed emotions around the event, and began to apply the Don't Want/Do Want exercise, the surface-level symptom – the pain – dissolved away and vanished.

My sister, who is a nurse practitioner, 'suddenly' developed type 1 diabetes in 2016 and was told she would have to inject insulin four times a day for the rest of her life. Looking beyond the illness, however, the eighteen months or so leading up to the diagnosis had been incredibly stressful and emotional, in ways too numerous to mention here, with one challenging situation following another, pushing her to physical and emotional breaking point. She had to keep going . . . but the diabetes diagnosis brought a dramatic shift in lifestyle and priorities.

What's interesting is what happened three years later, in 2019. As the previous stressful situations were resolved or left in the past, her life became happier, more relaxed and more peaceful. While away one weekend, her blood sugar suddenly dropped to levels that she felt were unsafe for injecting insulin, and remained that way for two weeks. She sought medical advice and was told that she no longer needed to inject as her insulin production had increased to levels greater than they had been at diagnosis.

At first her GP thought she had been misdiagnosed originally, but taking part in a major diabetes research programme, she had access to the UK's top experts in this, who confirmed her original diagnosis as being accurate but remained 'baffled' by her recovery. The doctors' working theory at the moment is that the stress of the year preceding onset had caused a massive build-up of cortisol (the hormone created by the threat response), which had impacted her autoimmune system, leading to a failing in the pancreas.

As life improved and stress reduced over the following years, her autoimmune system was allowed to return to normal and her pancreas began to produce more insulin. It's not perfect – probably around 25–50 per cent of what is considered normal – but it means that, at the time of writing, eighteen months later, she still has no need to inject and merely takes a pill to help her body use the insulin she does produce more efficiently. 'The more we know,' said her leading specialist, 'the more we realize we don't know.'

Our psychology affects our biology – and it can work either against us or for us. Most intelligent people will agree that a person's well-being is dependent upon a number of factors, including diet, exercise, lifestyle and psychology, and all these should really be taken into account when someone develops an illness.

While the work of pioneers like James Braid and Émile Coué has been around for more than a hundred years now, we still need more medical research in these areas in order to give medical practitioners the confidence to begin applying them more readily. One such area where some good research has been carried out is in the use of hypnotherapy visualization techniques for the treatment of IBS – irritable bowel syndrome – the condition referred to earlier in relation to the BBC *Horizon* documentary on placebos. Numerous studies have shown patients' ability to significantly reduce symptoms of pain, diarrhoea and bloating, as well as a reduction in the need for medication. In a practice exercise with a fellow student, one of my other students, who suffered with IBS, also managed to switch off her reaction to a certain food type, enabling her to take on some all-important energy she needed to complete some physical exercise she was involved in that day. Previously, she'd had to avoid the food type because of an adverse reaction.

If, as seems likely, we can combine these symptom-easing methods with looking *beyond the illness*, resolving any underlying causes owing to epigenetics and long-term stress through the threat response, as well as environmental factors, nutrition and sleep, the world of psychobiology and its role in recovery from illness is still very much an undiscovered country, one that has always intrigued and fascinated me.

PART FOUR

The Real You

Beyond the Clouds

I remember daydreamily staring out of the window one day – something I always seem to have been quite skilled at – desperately willing the clouds to part so that I could see the sun. And I remember it dawning on me in that moment that the sun is always there, always shining, but we often cannot see it because it is obscured by clouds.

Much of my therapeutic life I have spent helping people pull back their clouds to reveal their sunlight once again. Sunlight that was always there, just hidden, obscured or forgotten about. That sunlight is the Real You.

When most of us begin looking inside, asking who we are, what we are, and exploring our Inner Identity, what we often come across first are the clouds. The clouds seem real from a distance. Our fears, doubts and beliefs seem real from a distance.

So when we begin any kind of inner exploration, don't expect to find beautiful sunrises and sunsets, sun-kissed beaches with palm trees or whatever your own version of paradise might be. When we take a look inside what we usually come across first of all are more like storm clouds made up of fears, limitations and invisible beliefs – and when we poke around, we may even provoke an actual storm.

In real life this is where it can get scary, facing up to our feelings, emotions and beliefs. For some people it is just too much at first, so they would rather avoid this reality a while longer even though life will eventually catch up in one way or another. But when we can face the clouds of our own fears – and know that what we see is really an illusion created by beliefs picked up through our lifetime – and have the courage to get up close and examine them, then the illusion can begin to dissolve.

As I talked about earlier, clients often say to me, 'I am scared to find out who I really am. What if I really am horrible? What if I really am unlovable? What if I really am a despicable being?'

It is often much easier to turn away, back into the world, and start busying ourselves with whatever it is we do on the outside to make us feel temporarily better on the inside. But for anyone brave enough to peek beyond the clouds, the sun is most definitely shining – and our real, authentic, natural self is there, waiting, enjoying the warmth.

Over the years, it has become apparent to me that the majority of the fear-based ideas I have held about myself have turned out to be false. And the majority of fear-based ideas that my clients or students have held about themselves have also turned out to be false. It is a reasonable assumption that the same is therefore true for you as well – the majority of the fear-based ideas you hold about yourself are false, but they seem real.

It is important to understand this because when we start exploring inwardly and meet some stormy clouds, we need to know that, however real they may seem, they are not. When you can see beyond the clouds of your fears and find the Real You, you can feel peace, and all those things you have been chasing on the outside suddenly seem a little less important.

What You Really, Really Want

Earlier on we did an exercise and I said that what you really wanted from anything in life was an increase in one or more of your core beliefs.

- More 'enoughness'
- More safety and security
- More control
- More acceptance and connection
- More pleasure in love and relationships
- More en-lightenment

But even these are only stepping stones. What you really, really want is what having all this will give you.

What you really, really want is a deep sense of peace.

- Desire for more 'enoughness' => peace
- Desire for safety => peace
- Desire for more control => peace
- Desire for more acceptance and connection => peace
- More love and pleasure in relationships => peace
- A greater sense of en-lightenment => peace

In each and every moment, all we ever really want is a deep sense of peace.

With peace we can feel happiness; with peace we can encourage good health or come to terms with struggling health. Peace can bring us wealth, in the many meanings of the word; and peace can help us make better, more informed choices, compared to when we are running around like a stressed-out lunatic. Peace can leave us with space for ourselves, and space for others.

All we ever really want is peace.

That is something we can control and measure, moment by moment, day by day, and whatever plans life has in store for us, above all else, we can still choose peace.

Does this mean we just sit around meditating all day? No, of course not. Peace will come in many forms and there are many ways to get glimpses from our external world. For some it may be a skydive or riding a perfect wave; for others it may be the success of an exam or a business deal; for others still it may be a job well done, praise and adulation, or that satisfaction of a tasty meal, time spent with a loved one, playing an instrument, scoring a goal or an addiction to drink, drugs or sex. All can provide peace for a moment – but all will pass.

However, as we resolve our inner feelings and emotions, as we dissolve old fears and limiting beliefs about who we are and what we are, as we allow old identities to fall away and the new, more fulfilling Real You to take their place . . . that sense of peace expands more and more, into more areas of daily life.

Do we need to give up skydiving, surfing, being successful, receiving praise, enjoying good food, having loving relationships, drinking, getting high or having sex? Of course not. It just means we don't *need* to do those things to escape the bad or mundane and feel peace. We feel peace anyway, and then go and do those things, if we want to.

When we can stop trying to avoid the feelings created by the limitations of our fears and conditioning, and instead go beyond and begin to choose peace, our external world then seems to naturally reflect that. Our thoughts, feelings and behaviours become more constructive and when we do take part in the physical activities of the world, we do so through a more conscious choice for pleasure – which tends to be longer lasting.

All we ever really want is peace.

I mention this now because when we talk of letting go of an old identity we often associate this with a sense of loss or sacrifice. I tormented myself with this for many, many years. There were things I wanted – out there – that I thought would bring me peace – but the more I chased them, the more peace seemed to elude me.

I did stuff. I achieved stuff. I had some successes. I had some failures. Lots of them. But none of it ever lasted. None of it ever brought me any sense of lasting peace. Still, to give up on the idea of those dreams was unacceptable . . . I didn't want to just sit around doing nothing, achieving nothing, so I would try again and again. But the only thing that has ever truly brought me a lasting sense of peace is letting go of old ideas and limitations – layer by layer, feeling by feeling, belief by belief – and realizing that all we ever really want is peace, and so that is now my goal.

In any situation, I just want peace.

Each time I have done this, my level of peace has gone up a notch. And my level of happiness has increased a notch. And then when I do venture back out into the world, I do so with an increased sense of self-acceptance, freedom and peace with myself.

Some of this has happened in quite intensive E.S.C.A.P.E. therapy sessions, the type I do with clients; some of this has happened gradually, through the application of the ideas presented here, and others not yet mentioned. Other times it has been through 'life' itself forcing me to choose peace! But one thing that has made a world of difference is ending the attack – on myself and others – and finding ways to reinforce the five core beliefs.

I am good enough
I am safe and secure
I am strong, powerful and in control of myself
I am accepted and belong
I experience love as pleasure
And, above all else, all I really want
is peace

Summary

So here is the situation that each of us face, as I see it.

We are born into this world and it appears that stuff happens to us. Some of it feels good, some of it doesn't, but whatever it is, it shapes and forms our beliefs which we then carry with us through life, further shaping and moulding our lives and experiences.

Although it seems on one level that life happens to us, there is a strong possibility or probability that we are actually both creating and experiencing life simultaneously, according to our beliefs and conditioning, with free will battling away in between.

Any time we choose, we can update those beliefs and conditioning, but as much of it occurs subconsciously, we do not believe we can.

Challenging these can cause fear and anger, via the threat response, as a resistance to change – remember, all resistance is fear.

And yet at the same time, the whole system seems designed to keep providing us with opportunities to face our fears, or the effects of them, driving us to evolve and become something more.

Underneath all of our anxieties and limiting beliefs, however, there is actually a lighter, freer version of our self – the Real You – one who is deeply at peace with himself or herself, lives in the moment and is a gift to the world around them.

And the moment we can begin to acknowledge that – and work with it – life begins to take on a new meaning and many of the physical and emotional struggles of life we have been through can begin to ease or dissolve away.

But the real pain of life is a resistance to that change – and the various 'letting gos' that entails. With every letting go of an old idea or belief, we escape the limitations of our lives – many of which were far more self-imposed than we realized – and as we become more and more self-realized, we can finally become more of the person we were born to be.

Reading this was the easy bit. But now you know, you can never go back.

You can pretend to forget for a while like I have done numerous times . . . but you can never go back, and eventually you will begin to remember.

You will always know that whatever you experience, somewhere, somehow, in some way, every moment is an opportunity to either repeat an old pattern or evolve into something new. There is always a choice to give away your power or to use it; to remain stuck or to evolve; to stay trapped or to E.S.C.A.P.E.

It is possible to do this by yourself if you are persistent and brave; but very often an experienced professional or helpful Escape Buddy will be able to speed up the process for you by helping you make the invisible visible and reflecting it back to you. But never worry about being left behind – life will always be nudging you in the right direction, in the right way, at the right time.

On a deeper level still, who are we really? Are we just these biophysical blobs of mostly water, randomly firing neurons and chemicals, bumbling our way through life, having random experiences with no meaning or significance, which just happened to evolve out of previous versions of the same, as many would have us believe? Or are we something more profound than that? In *The Nature of Personal Reality*, Jane Roberts wrote:

> You are given the gift of the gods
> You create your reality according to your beliefs.
> Yours is the creative energy that makes your world
> There are no limitations to the self except those you believe in.

For now, I'll leave it to you to decide! But, based on my own experience and studying the minds of thousands of clients over nearly thirty years . . . I know which one makes the most sense to me.

We have talked of core fears, beliefs, conditioning and the threat response as being at the root cause of all our personal, emotional and habitual problems, and possibly many of our physical ills as well. We look out on the world or form images in our mind and see danger, threat and attack – or the potential for it. What we really want is to move away from a fear-based version of ourselves and towards a more natural, authentically real version, to feel at peace with ourselves and at peace with the world and all in it.

Therefore, as one final exercise, wherever you are, whoever you are with and whatever you are doing, if ever you find yourself feeling any kind of distress . . .

**Take a breath . . .
Clear your mind . . .
And remind yourself . . .
All I really want here . . . is peace.**

The Next Step

The next step is up to you, but if you want something to change you have to do something about it and I'd love to help you with that.

If you are interested in finding out more, start by going to andrew-parr.com and check out the resources we have created for you.

If you'd like some extra one-to-one help to break through some of those fears and limitations, you can book sessions with one of our trained, licensed practitioners.

We do also offer the opportunity to become a practitioner with us at our academy, and if you would like to transform your own life by helping others escape the limitations of theirs, you can begin here, where we have created some free initial training for you, to make sure we are a good fit: www.andrew-parr.com/frectraining

Whichever next step feels right for you, do drop by and say hi, or ask a question, because in one way or another we are all in this together and it would be great to hear from you: hello@andrew-parr.com

With warm wishes,
Andrew Parr

Some Thank Yous

To my biological parents, Gloria and Roy, for bringing me into the world and having the courage to do what you had to do.

To my mum and dad, Gill and Brian, for choosing me in the clinic that day, loving me, bringing me up and giving me a good life filled with opportunities.

To the Wilsmores, Wards, Joneses, Jonah Wails and Baldwin/Woods for welcoming me into their respective families at different times in my life.

To my sister Lynne and her husband Neil for always being there.

To John James for giving me a Plan For Life.

To Neil French, Georges Philips and Walter Broadbent for being my first hypno teachers, and to Dave Elman and Gil Boyne for deepening my knowledge.

To Jane Roberts and the 'Seth' books for helping my mind boldly go where it may not have gone otherwise.

To Jani King and the 'P'taah' books for introducing me to the four fears and allowing me to teach them.

To the numerous people who have helped me unpick my own madness.

To the students, graduates and clients who have also been my teachers, and especially those who were brave enough to let me share their stories.

To everyone at Penguin for their invaluable help at every stage of putting this book together – I had no idea how much work goes into it!

To my children – Alice, Milo and Alfie – for teaching *me* right from wrong, giving me a reason to exist, at a time when I couldn't see one in myself, and for all the fun and laughter, before and since.

I love you loads, thanks for everything, and apologies for any way in which I have messed up as a dad! At least this book should help you know how to put it right!

And finally, to Alison, my partner, best friend and mother of our children, for picking me up when I was low, pulling me down when I was lost in the clouds, keeping me sane, grounded, loved, inspired and, most importantly, fed and supplied with cake! I don't think I could have done it without you, and wouldn't have wanted to anyway. Here's to the next chapter!

Index

Page references in *italics* indicate images.

Index